Praise for **Compassion for**

"Stunning revelations. Michelle Becker's approach has helped us find a deeper connection and finally stop trying to fix each other—paradoxically, by learning to be kind to ourselves. The 'Core Values' exercise yanked us out of the routine doldrums of marriage and reminded us why we are together. We are grateful."

—*Becky and Tim P., Fort Wayne, Indiana*

"This beautiful book will help couples move their relationships from a place of pain and blame to love and acceptance. Drawing on empirically supported self-compassion practices, the author provides concrete tools to help people open their hearts to themselves so they can open fully to their partners."

—*Kristin Neff, PhD, coauthor of* The Mindful Self-Compassion Workbook

"The absorbing, step-by-step approach makes the exercises easy to dive into. I especially enjoyed the 'Touching Hands' exercise, where my partner and I experienced what it felt like to withdraw or be withdrawn from. This is definitely the book for anyone who wants to break negative relationship patterns and work toward the love you deserve."

—*Lynn H., Pleasanton, California*

"From her vast experience as a therapist and teacher, Michelle Becker has written a masterpiece for any couple, whether you are seeking greater intimacy or help with serious conflicts. Her advice is grounded in science, with lots of examples and many simple, powerful exercises. Beautiful, timely, and important."

—*Rick Hanson, PhD, author of* Resilient

"We would all like to have relationships that are constantly supportive, empathic, and fun—but, unfortunately, things don't always work out that way. Having compassion for each other allows us to resolve conflicts, face disappointments, accept compromise, and learn the arts of apology and forgiveness. For anyone interested in building relationships based on courage, wisdom, and deep friendship, this is an ideal, inspiring guide."

—*Paul Gilbert, PhD, FBPsS, OBE, author of* The Compassionate Mind

"Michelle Becker is the therapist any couple would be lucky to find when they hit a rough spot—she is wise, practical, and without judgment. *Compassion for Couples* will transform your relationship."

—*Susan M. Pollak, MTS, EdD, author of* Self-Compassion for Parents

Compassion for Couples

Compassion for Couples

Building the Skills
of Loving Connection

Michelle Becker

Foreword by Christopher Germer

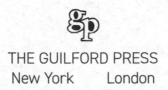

THE GUILFORD PRESS
New York   London

Copyright © 2023 The Guilford Press
A Division of Guilford Publications, Inc.
370 Seventh Avenue, Suite 1200, New York, NY 10001
www.guilford.com

The information in this volume is not intended as a substitute for
consultation with healthcare professionals. Each individual's health concerns
should be evaluated by a qualified professional.

See page 276 for terms of use for audio files.

Printed in the United States of America

Last digit is print number: 9   8   7   6   5   4   3   2   1

Library of Congress Cataloging-in-Publication Data is available from the
publisher.

ISBN 978-1-4625-4515-5 (paperback) — ISBN 978-1-4625-5057-9 (hardcover)

Contents

Part I
Start Where You Are
Understanding How Things Go Wrong in Relationships
and How Things Get Better

v

Part II

Building a Foundation for Compassion in Your Relationship

Mindfulness, Common Humanity, and Kindness

Part III

Putting It into Practice

Tailoring Compassion Skills to Your Relationship

Purchasers of this book can download audio files of select exercises at *www.guilford.com/becker2-materials* or on the author's website at *https://wisecompassion.com/cfcbookaudios* for personal use or use with clients (see copyright page for details).

List of Exercises

---

*An audio recording of this exercise is available. See the List of Audio Tracks.

Foreword

It's an honor to write a foreword to this groundbreaking book by Michelle Becker. Michelle is a talented marriage and family therapist, a seasoned mindfulness teacher, and a leader in the emerging field of compassion training. I had the privilege of teaching Michelle's compassion for couples course with her, and I personally experienced its depth and beauty. As a clinical psychologist and couples therapist, I'm also aware of the traps that couples can fall into and how difficult it can be to get out of them. In this book, Michelle lays out her innovative approach in the clearest of terms and gets right to the heart of the matter—helping couples.

Burgeoning research shows that compassion is a powerful resource. Compassion increases happiness and life satisfaction, decreases stress and anxiety, enhances physical health and well-being, and, most importantly for this book, improves our relationships. Compassion is also multidimensional. It can be directed toward others or toward ourselves (self-compassion). Compassion can be soft or strong. Usually we think of compassion as soft and tender, but isn't standing up to unfairness with a firm "No!" also a form of compassion? Michelle unpacks the many nuances of compassion and shows how they can be applied, safely and effectively, to enhance intimate relationships.

I'm a big fan of Michelle's positive, nonpathological approach to working with couples. When couples are struggling, the last thing they need is to focus on the flaws they perceive in one another. Instead, compassion is all about acceptance and care. This doesn't mean that we're supposed to accept unacceptable behavior, or force ourselves to care, or give up on the idea of change. Rather, compassion puts the change agenda on a different footing—radical acceptance. As the psychologist Carl Rogers wrote, "the curious paradox is that when I accept myself as I am . . . change seems to come about almost unnoticed." The same goes for our partners. When they feel accepted, they're more likely to change. Readers who have tried in vain to change "sticky" patterns in their relationships might be ready for this new approach.

Acceptance is not always easy to come by in relationships. After all, our partners are conditioned human beings, just like ourselves, with likes and dislikes. And the most difficult person to accept is usually ourselves. Research shows that most people are more compassionate toward others than themselves. Fortunately, self-compassion can be practiced and learned. When we're struggling, we can ask ourselves the question, "What do I need?" If we need acceptance, we can learn to accept ourselves. If we need validation, we can validate ourselves. We're not giving up on getting what we need from our partners. Rather, self-compassion increases the likelihood that our partners will accept us as we are and meet our needs because there's less pressure to do so.

Michelle is a leading expert on self-compassion. She has contributed substantially to the mindful self-compassion (MSC) curriculum, which has been taught to over 250,000 people around the world. Typically, near the end of an MSC course, participants are eager to apply self-compassion to the challenges in their lives. One of the most common questions is "How can I bring self-compassion into the relationship with my partner?" This book brilliantly answers that question. For example, everything that works in relationship to yourself can be extended to your partner. If you ask yourself, "What do I need?" you can also ask your partner, "What do *you* need?" If you want to live in harmony with your core values and you would like your partner to support your efforts, you can also inquire about your partner's core values and how you might support *their* efforts. I experienced this process firsthand, and it works like magic to bring couples together.

Another unique aspect of Michelle's model is how she has blended MSC with compassion-focused therapy (CFT). MSC and CFT are the two most widely disseminated compassion training programs in the world today. At the heart of CFT is an awareness of motivational systems that underlie all we say and do. We can be motivated to avoid a threat, to achieve a goal, or to connect and care. Each motivational system has its own physiology. Generally speaking, when we feel threatened, or have the goal of changing our partners, the interaction will end in frustration. However, when we're in a caring frame of mind, whatever we say or do is likely to bring a positive outcome. As Michelle says, "It's more about the state we're in than the words we use." This book shows us how to cultivate a caring and compassionate state of mind with our intimate partner, often the most challenging person in our lives!

There is no couple relationship without challenges. As family therapist Salvador Minuchin quipped, "Every marriage is a mistake; it's how you deal with it that matters." Compassion is probably the wisest option for dealing with difficulties in a relationship. Compassion assumes that we're all imperfect human beings, we all make mistakes, we all suffer, and we all wish to be free from suffering. Compassion gives us an opportunity to address our relationship problems from a position of common humanity. As you read this book, you'll notice how fair the author is to both members of the couple, not favoring one over the other, while offering valuable tools to address the inevitable challenges.

This book is designed to help couples heal and thrive. Compassion does both. Compassion is a positive emotion. It brings energy and happiness into our lives. Therefore, when we wrap ourselves and our partners in compassion, suffering is transformed into something different, even into joy. It's like alchemy, but it has to be personally experienced to be understood. Please go ahead and try, and see what happens in your own relationship.

CHRISTOPHER GERMER, PhD
Harvard Medical School

Acknowledgments

This book is proof of the truth of our interconnection and interdependence. Although the words and ideas are mine, they would not have come to be without the support and influence of countless others throughout my lifetime. And beyond my own lifetime, I want to acknowledge the lineage of teachers through time: my teachers, those who have influenced my teachers, and the teachers of my teachers. I am merely a conduit for the wisdom and compassion they unfolded, and it is my hope that the benefits of these concepts and practices will flow to you in whatever way you find most helpful. Any mistakes are mine alone, and any benefits are surely due to the collective wisdom and compassion of those who have walked before and beside me.

My parents, Marilyn and John (Mom and Dad to me), were my first teachers and shaped my personality. Thank you for loving me all my life.

I am grateful to have friends who've known me most of my life, with whom I still gather as often as possible: Laura, Lauren, Lina, Lynn (P. L.), and Colleen. You knew who I was before I did, and through you I discovered my own goodness.

There have also been those who taught me well and gave me confidence along the way, including my teachers, mentors, supervisors, and colleagues in undergraduate and graduate school, and in my work as a marriage and family therapist. You know who you are. Thank you!

Those who have nurtured me along the way by holding space for me as difficult feelings arose and who reassured me that all was well, even when things fell apart, are especially dear to me. The capacity to dive deeply into the nature of my own suffering has been the greatest teacher for me. Through this, I've been able to find a groundedness in the midst of difficulty and an openheartedness to those who are suffering. It has given me the capacity to understand the nature of suffering and to accompany those in its midst. As you held space for me, you gave me the capacity to hold space for others.

Over the years, I've been held and supported by the teachings of many teachers, especially Sylvia Boorstein, Tara Brach, Pema Chödrön, Roshi Joan Halifax, Thich Nhat Hanh, Thupten Jinpa, Wendy Johnson, Jack Kornfield, H. H. the Dalai Lama, Joanna Macy, Sharon Salzberg, and Gina Sharpe. Deep bow of gratitude to each of you. To Frank Ostaseski, whose teaching touches my heart deeply and inspires and supports my practice, endless gratitude.

To my friends and colleagues who encouraged (and at times shoved) me into the role of teaching compassion and then teaching teachers how to teach compassion, thank you for all of it, especially the laughs and joy along the way. To Steve Hickman, who encouraged me to teach mindfulness-based stress reduction at the University of California San Diego (UCSD) Center for Mindfulness, encouraged me to pursue mindful self-compassion (MSC), and then became my constant companion on the journey, thank you for always making sure I am entertained and for keeping the motor running. Chris Germer and Kristin Neff, who recognized the fruits of my practice, invited me to help hone the MSC program and codevelop (along with Steve Hickman) the MSC teacher training, valued my contributions, blew my mind and softened my heart with their teachings, and always encouraged me to offer my gifts to the world. For your friendship, your teachings, and especially your encouragement and support as I developed the Compassion for Couples (CFC) program—not the least of which was encouraging me to use the MSC program as my jumping-off point—deep, deep appreciation and gratitude.

To my Compassion Cultivation Training (CCT) teacher trainers—Erika Rosenberg, Margaret Cullen, Monica Hanson, Leah Weiss, and Kelly McGonigal—thank you for diving deeply into the pedagogy of compassion as you skillfully embodied compassion. And to my CCT colleagues—you know who you are—I count myself lucky to be a part of such a wonderful community.

I am especially grateful for the sisterhood of compassion teachers and dear friends to whom I can always turn for understanding, advice, and support, especially Susan Pollak, Beth Mulligan, and Dawn Mac-Donald. You keep me grounded and inspired. I count myself lucky to be in your midst. And to the group of colleagues who supported each other in mentorship: Tina Gibson, Vanessa Hope, Judith Soulsby, Christine Braehler, Dawn MacDonald, and Susan Pollak. You were each so much wiser than you knew, and your vulnerability and compassion left a lasting imprint on me. I'm grateful for all we learned together.

To my friends and colleagues at the UCSD Center for Mindfulness, especially the original team: Lorraine Hobbs, Noriko Harth, Livia Walsh, Megan Prager, Sara Schairer, Renee Lewis, Luis Morones, Allen Goldstein, Deborah Rana, and Steve Hickman. It has been a pleasure to work together.

I also want to acknowledge and appreciate Lorri Hilbert, with whom I cofounded the San Diego Center for Well Being and alongside whom I learned and taught the Daring Way™; and Cassondra Graff, with whom I explored and practiced integrating mindfulness skills into psychotherapy for couples. It was a pleasure to learn and collaborate with each of you.

A bow of gratitude to those who have lent their expertise to the development of the CFC program along the way: Sean Cook, for his early collaboration; Pittman McGehee, for his co-teaching and friendship—it always made me smile to teach with you, Pittman; Aimee Eckhardt, for her mad tech skills, encouragement, suggestions, and depth; Ann Bowles, for her talent, support, and friendship; and Megan Prager, my friend and current CFC co-teacher. And the research team at Florida State University: Myriam Rudaz, Thomas Ledermann, Amelia Welch, and Greg Seibert. I love your creativity, dedication, and insights.

There are those who have generously shared their experiences with me, especially my patients, from whom I have learned more than I ever knew possible, and my students in the various courses

I've taught, especially CFC. You have been my teachers, and I've been deeply moved by your courage, vulnerability, and resilience. Thank you for trusting me. I carry your stories with me.

Each person listed, in their own way, helped to develop the foundation for this book—and for that and so much more I am grateful.

A special group of people supported the writing of this book, most notably:

Kirsten Ritter, who eagerly read every chapter, skillfully suggested edits, and has been instrumental in getting *Compassion for Couples* out into the world. Your enthusiasm and kindness is sincerely appreciated. Thank you.

Lorraine Hobbs, friend, colleague, and writing buddy, whose insight and friendship are greatly appreciated. Thank you for believing in me, writing alongside me, and listening to my writing week after week. Your support and encouragement was definitely a highlight of this process, and I can't imagine writing this book without you.

My very talented editors and the team at The Guilford Press, especially Kitty Moore (Publisher, General Trade), who believed in the book and encouraged me to write, all the while steering the book in the right direction (over and over again), and Christine Benton (Developmental Editor), whose keen eye and talented edits were ever present in service of making this book a good experience for readers. This book is vastly better for their involvement. I am grateful for your talent, dedication, and hard work (lots of it!). I especially appreciate the way you both came along with me as I told my stories and your instincts to stick up for me when I described the various challenges that arose for me. You are a compassionate team!

My family was the bright spot throughout this process. My now grown children have taught me the meaning of love and compassion. Words can't express how proud I am of each of you, and what a gift you are in my world. I've learned so much from each of you. It's been such a pleasure to be your mom.

And my dear husband, Steve, to whom I've been married for thirty-eight years now. Our marriage has been the biggest training ground for compassion in couples as we've moved through our own three stages of relationships. Even when I'm hunkered down writing, I know you're always in my corner. Thank you for all the love, foot rubs, tech support, meal prep, encouragement, and believing in me. Your love and support on so many levels have made this book possible.

May all beings find the joy of loving and being loved.

* * *

The following publishers have generously given permission to reprint material from copyrighted works:

From "Kindness" in *Words Under the Words: Selected Poems*, by Naomi Shihab Nye. Copyright © 1995. Used with permission of Far Corner Books.

From *The Book of Awakening* (20th anniv. ed.), by Mark Nepo. Copyright © 2020 Mark Nepo. Used by permission of Red Wheel/ Weiser.

From "Prayer Before the Prayer" in *The Book of Forgiving*, by Desmond Tutu and Mpho Tutu. Copyright © 2014 Desmond M. Tutu and Mpho A. Tutu. Used by permission of HarperCollins Publishers and HarperCollins Publishers, Ltd.

From "Hold Out Your Hand" in *Staying in Love*, by Julia Fehrenbacher. Copyright © 2021 Julia Fehrenbacher. Reprinted by permission of the author.

Introduction

In my personal and professional experience, I've been astounded by the power of relationships to wound and to heal us. There is nothing quite as heartbreaking as longing to be loved and feeling unloved. And there is nothing quite as heartwarming as feeling seen, accepted, and loved just as we are. It is even more heartbreaking when we've found a relationship that feels healing and then turns into a source of distress. We wonder what went wrong. Is there something wrong with me? Am I just unlovable? Is there something wrong with my partner? Most often, even if we have an underlying doubt that we are lovable, we set our sights on what is wrong with our partners. It's not that we *want* something to be wrong with them—quite the opposite. It's just that we've tried everything we know how to try and we hope that if we point out their faults they'll change and become the partners we were hoping for. Perhaps the partners we thought we had. It's a really common strategy—one that is often unconscious. Yet in doing so we're placing all of the power in our partners' hands rather than our own. Even though things would be easier if our partners showed up in ways that helped us feel safe and loved, we can still change the patterns in our relationships by changing our own side of the equation.

What might happen if instead of getting caught in this downward relationship spiral we paused for a moment and took the time to understand what was really going on? Not at the surface of things where reactivity plays with us, but down deeper where we begin to understand the terrain of relationships and how our wiring leads us astray? In my work with couples, this is a pivotal moment. When people really begin to understand that these issues and patterns are normal and it is more about our stress responses than about how much we love each other, relief floods their bodies. And the door to hope opens up.

From Falling in Love to Mature Love

There is a normal trajectory for relationships. In the first phase, what I might call the "falling in love" phase, our bodies are flooded with a hormonal cocktail that infuses us with happiness. At this stage we often feel like we've found the missing link in life. That our partners have brought happiness into our lives. We can only see the good in each other and believe that this other person is responsible for our happiness. Fairy tales always stop here, followed by the phrase "and they lived happily ever after." Only that isn't what typically happens in real life. This first phase of love is important; the hormones help us attach and bond with another human being, which can feel wonderful. But alas, this cocktail wears off eventually.

Then we enter the second phase, where we notice and often fixate on the undesirable qualities in our partners—those seemingly small annoyances that, over time, build into bigger resentments. Maybe, like one of the couples you'll meet in this book, you find yourselves arguing over things like how to load the dishwasher—and then learn that such apparent trivialities are really a sign of the distress each of you has been feeling in the relationship. Or perhaps you have blowups about who is doing more for the family that end up pushing you apart when what you both need is a compassionate response to your needs. When we get caught in this cycle of reactivity, over time it chips away at our connection and love until we feel great distress in the relationship and start to wonder how we missed these now glaring flaws in our partners. What started as undesirable qualities now seem like character flaws, and we wonder if the relationship is doomed. Sometimes we turn away from each other in an effort to avoid conflict, and this too creates more distance in our relationships. To make matters worse, life deals us inevitable challenges, even if those challenges are positive and desired, like the stress of raising children and building careers. Of course, our challenges aren't limited to the positive and desired; we also find ourselves challenged by hardships in life. All of this can have us fearing that our relationship is doomed when it so recently felt like the answer to our prayers.

It is at this very time that pausing and taking a deeper look at what is really happening can help us understand and accept ourselves and our partners. We can learn mindfulness and compassion skills that can become the habits of tending to our own needs, offering support to our partners, fostering intimacy, and deepening and solidifying our connection. Building skills specific to ourselves, our partners, and our relationships can provide a solid road map for how to meet ourselves and our partners with compassion, rather than fall into patterns of reactivity that are rooted in old physiology designed to keep us safe—and which actually wreak havoc on our relationships.

Mindfulness, as we explore it in the context of relationships, has two beneficial aspects. First, it helps us step out of reactivity and take an honest look at where we are and what we need. Second, it is a resource we can use to steady ourselves any time we begin to feel pulled into reactivity and overwhelm. This allows us to show up in our relationships having cultivated wisdom rather than being pushed around by reactivity.

Compassion is a way of meeting ourselves and our partners with kindness—especially when things aren't going well for us—right when we most need it. When we learn to direct our kindness toward ourselves—in other words, to use self-compassion—we are no longer dependent on our partners for comforting and soothing. We have what we need exactly when we need it. This really changes everything. Knowing that we have what we need, especially when times get rough, especially if no one else shows up for us, gives us the courage to face what is arising in ourselves, our partners, and our relationships. With self-compassion we can comfort and soothe ourselves when we need it and we have the strength to set limits and boundaries with kindness as needed. We can risk becoming more vulnerable because we have a safety net of self-compassion should things not go well. And when we are vulnerable, it is much easier for our partners to come closer to us.

Because we learn to meet our partners with compassion when

they are caught in distress (including reactivity), they begin to feel safer with us as well. They can risk being vulnerable too. And that's key, because there is no intimacy without vulnerability. How could we possibly feel loved if we don't let our partners know who we truly are? Rather than covering ourselves with protective shields, when we build compassion into our relationships we can really let our guard down. Then we can come closer and develop a truly satisfying relationship.

These mindfulness and compassion skills form the basis for moving your relationship out of the often painful second phase of relationships and into the third phase, which I'll call "mature love." In this phase we are more fully ourselves *and* more solidly connected. These relationships are characterized by acceptance as much as they are by a deep sense of love. Whereas in the first phase there is connection, but we don't see ourselves or our partners clearly, in the mature phase we are more fully ourselves and the connection is more solid. The path to this mature love phase often involves that difficult second phase, and that's what this book is about—how we can learn and use mindfulness and compassion skills in relationships to meet our own needs, support each other, and grow into the relationship we want.

Of course, you don't have to be struggling with a painful relationship to use this book. In my psychotherapy practice with couples, I've found compassion training is *the* thing that best helps couples develop this foundation of caring in relationships and move into the mature love phase in which we feel seen, accepted, loved, and secure. Compassion is also *the* thing that will deepen and solidify your already satisfying relationship so that it stands the test of time.

My Professional Path

When I became a licensed marriage and family therapist (LMFT), I found the career path full of heart for me—it was the path that put the importance of relationships front and center. I worked with people as young as four and as old as ninety-four and was taken by the power of relationships throughout our lives. But the most satisfying work for me has been my work with couples. Most therapists will tell you couples therapy is more challenging. Early on in my work with couples I did find it more challenging. Even though my work was grounded in the theories of the day, I found treatment wasn't as successful with couples as I'd hoped. Even when I'd had a "success" with a couple in session, they often found it difficult to maintain between our sessions. One or another thing would happen, and they'd find themselves caught in a pattern of reactivity again.

Around this time I discovered mindfulness. I loved the way it fostered wisdom by helping people see more clearly and decreased the potential to be hijacked by reactivity. It was on a mindfulness retreat that I discovered self-compassion. In mindfulness and self-compassion training I learned what I now teach—how to relate to *experiences* with more wisdom and less reactivity and how to relate to *myself and others* with more kindness and understanding.

Drs. Christopher Germer and Kristen Neff, the developers of mindful self-compassion (MSC), invited me to begin teaching their course. Then, in 2014, Drs. Germer, Neff, Steve Hickman, and I codeveloped the MSC teacher training, and it was on one of these MSC teacher trainings that I conceived of the idea of adapting the MSC curriculum for use with couples. My interest was twofold. First, so much suffering was happening in people's primary relationships, and I saw a clear path to alleviating that suffering. Second, applying compassion training to our primary relationships takes us beyond the alleviation of suffering and into the territory of having a safe place from which we can grow as people, become more fully ourselves, and find our place in the larger scheme of things. We can take risks and go for what our heart desires because we have a soft place to land.

When I ran the idea by Drs. Germer and Neff, they immediately encouraged me to pursue the venture and authorized the use of the MSC curriculum in developing the curriculum for couples. Eventually I developed the Compassion for Couples (CFC) program and began teaching it to couples in 2017. While the program has its roots in the MSC program, it goes beyond self-compassion in training how to use that as the base to then move into practicing compassion for our partners, and building a secure foundation of kindness and compassion in our relationships.

From the beginning I've been amazed at the power of the CFC program to transform relationships. Participants have reported a renewed sense of warmth, gratitude, friendliness, and safety in their relationships; a lot more mutual understanding and kindness; and new communication skills that enriched their lives together. Some discovered that compassion had put their relationships—always so important to them—back in the center of their lives. Many have been surprised at how quickly these new skills can improve their relationships.

Even more touching for me are the comments from couples who already had healthy relationships. These couples remarked on how the course has strengthened their relationships and allowed them to show more of themselves to their partners. They too felt more connected than ever before. And it has been especially sweet to work with engaged couples, whose work set them on the path to a long and satisfying relationship, even when difficulties arise.

The CFC program has been honed over many cohorts with the input of my co-teachers and collaborators and mostly from the feedback from couples themselves. Research is currently under way through Florida State University.

About This Book

For whatever reason, you may not have the ability to take the CFC course with your partner. That's why I wrote this book. I want you to have access to the mindfulness and compassion skills that can help you find your way into the mature love phase of relationships. I want to help you uncover where things go awry when you and your partner get caught in reactivity. To see this in the context of what happens when our wiring for survival gets activated, and how it trips us up in relationships. How our efforts to get out of pain often create more pain. I'd like to help you see these things through the eyes of compassion, because that really changes our experience. Most of all, I want to help you build a system of care into your relationships. Care for yourself *and* care for your partner and relationship. What most of us want from each other is a kind and loving presence above all else.

This book is filled with exercises and other opportunities for you to find and strengthen those qualities that foster the tools within you that will lead you to a more satisfying way of being in your relationship.

With these tools, you'll grow in your capacity for compassion, for yourself and your partner. And then you'll go beyond fostering your own skills and learn how to personalize compassion based on what you, your partner, and your relationship need the most. When these concepts become practices, and these practices turn into habits, our relationships become infused with love. And that changes everything.

This book comes out of the CFC program, and many of the exercises are from the program. Additionally, many of the exercises in the CFC program come out of the MSC program, though most have been adapted for use with couples. I want to honor and acknowledge my friends and colleagues Drs. Germer and Neff and the Center for MSC for their permission to use the MSC practices and for their skill in developing the MSC program. MSC is an empirically supported and effective program for learning self-compassion. I recommend it wholeheartedly and have put information about the program and various ways to learn self-compassion in the Resources section of this book. MSC and CFC, each stand-alone programs, are highly complementary.

The stories in this book come from my experience with couples in psychotherapy, in teaching, and in life. To protect the confidentiality of these couples, and to illustrate the concepts most clearly, the stories are an amalgamation of couples, and the names have been changed. I have learned a tremendous amount from them, and I think you will too.

This book is for everyone regardless of age, socioeconomic status, education level, race and ethnicity, gender identity, sexual orientation; regardless of whatever phase of relationship you are in; whether you are in distress and needing to find your way back to what is healing and healthy, or happy together and wanting to build a solid foundation for the future. Whether you are in a new relationship or have been together for decades. To get the most out of this book, it helps to be in a committed relationship. Please know that this book is not a substitute for psychotherapy and when there are issues of substance abuse, domestic violence (physical or emotional), or infidelity, these issues often need to be resolved before engaging in relationship work. A good therapist can be especially helpful in these situations. Stability and safety take priority.

How to Use the Book

Throughout the book, there are explanations, stories, and practices to help you understand the concepts and skills, but even more so to apply them to your own situation and develop practices and habits that support you and your relationship. By engaging in the "Try This" exercises, you can move the understanding from your head to your heart. It isn't the theory of compassion that is helpful; rather it is the practice of compassion that brings the associated benefits. Applying what you learn, as you are learning it, anchors the learning more deeply and can really be motivating to develop your compassion practices.

You may find it helpful to have a journal to use to record your responses to the exercises, as well as to note important concepts that you would like to remember. You can also follow along with audio tracks I've provided for some of the practices in the exercises (see the List of Audio Tracks at the end of the book) For ease of practice, some of these exercises are combined into a single audio. While it is ideal when both partners read the book and do the exercises, it isn't required for you and your relationships to benefit. Like me, when you work on your own compassion practice, it is bound to spill over into your relationship. It is my hope that this book makes fostering the skills of compassion in relationships available to all.

The book is organized into three parts. In Part I we begin by opening to and understanding where you are right now. I've adapted Paul Gilbert's work on emotion regulation systems to help you identify and understand your relational patterns, your partner's relational patterns, and how those patterns dance together. As you come to see these patterns, you will also come to understand how normal and human it is to get caught in these patterns of reactivity. And you will begin to glimpse how to free yourself.

In Part II we continue by exploring the foundations of compassion for self and other through the lens of mindfulness, common humanity, and kindness. This section helps to open the heart and build solid foundational bonds with your partner based in kindness, caring, and compassion.

In Part III we turn our attention to how to put these compassion skills into action in our relationships. While you can, of course, start anywhere you like in the book, you'll get the most benefit from the book by reading the parts in order. Just as when building a house, more stability comes from building a foundation of understanding, then erecting a structure of caring for each other, before putting on the roof of compassionate action.

Please keep in mind as you read that, whatever our differences, we are connected in our need to belong and to feel loved and connected. In my work teaching compassion, and in my psychotherapy work, I practice, as best I can, acceptance and inclusivity. I find that courses are better the more diversity is present in the room. It breaks my heart when patients tentatively work up the courage to tell me that they are gay or trans as they hold their breath wondering if they'll be accepted or rejected. And, of course, many people who have been marginalized don't feel comfortable speaking up at all. Whatever your experience of marginalization in the world, please know that here in these pages you are wanted and accepted just as you are. I've done my best to use pronouns, wording, and examples that are inclusive. (You'll find I alternate between the pronouns she, he, and they. Please feel free to switch out the pronoun in your mind to the correct pronoun for you.) Undoubtedly there will be places where I have failed to do so in some way. I apologize in advance for any commissions or omissions that make anyone feel they are not welcome or do not belong. It is my dream that everyone will come to know their value and realize they do belong. Whoever you are, you are wanted and welcome in these pages.

Part I

Start Where You Are

Understanding How Things Go Wrong
in Relationships
and How Things Get Better

The first five chapters of this book offer you an opportunity to open to and understand where you are in your relationship right now. You'll gain some great insights into how powerful reactivity is in relationships and why we all behave in ways we may not see clearly but use very reflexively. With an understanding of how often that reflexivity steers us wrong, you can begin to glimpse how you might take a different direction. You'll learn how to identify your relationship patterns, your partner's relationship patterns, and how those patterns dance together. As you come to understand these patterns, you will also start to see how normal and human it is to get caught in these patterns of reactivity. And you will begin to glimpse how to free yourself.

1

We All Need to Be Loved

Life is the flower for which love is the honey.
—VICTOR HUGO

The room was overflowing with kindness, connection, love. I felt the buzzing, at once stimulating and calming, enlivening. There was vulnerability, there was joy, sadness, forgiveness, longing. But most of all there was a palpable sense of love. Time stood still. It was one of those moments that seemed without beginning or end, the kind you were just happy to be in, without a drop of desire for anything else. "This is the *real* making love," Chris said. My eyes brimmed with tears and a lump formed in my throat. I could only nod in agreement. The moment took my breath away, the way the awe of turning a corner and finding an incredibly beautiful scenic vista takes the breath away.

It didn't begin like this. We were about twenty-four hours into a Compassion for Couples (CFC) program. My colleague, Chris Germer, and I had welcomed eleven couples to a quaint little inn in the mountains. We had a variety of couples, ones that had been together a long time, ones that were engaged, ones that were happily married, others that were unhappy, very unhappy. Couples who were older and those who were younger. Straight couples, gay couples, couples of varying ethnicity, color, and identities. None of those things mattered. What we shared was much more valuable. At the heart of things we all longed to be loved.

We had already opened to difficulty and imperfection. We'd opened to the ways we protect ourselves and our relationships and

13

how absolutely human that is. We'd explored how the ways we try to protect ourselves and our relationships can often cause real and lasting damage. We'd opened to our hurts and those of our loved ones. And, most of all, we'd opened to our own capacity to be kind in the face of pain and difficulty. To see and accept, even love, each other as we are—fully human, warts and all. And here we sat, Chris and I, in the midst of the courageous vulnerability of love, as we witnessed the sometimes long, dry thirst for a drop of love quenched, as words of kindness and love fell like raindrops from the sky. A gentle, warm rain. The kind that cleanses, nourishes, and satisfies the dry, parched earth. Our couples were whispering them to each other.

How did we get here? It wasn't easy. And yet it wasn't as hard as it seemed it might be, either. And we all knew the preciousness of it because we knew it wasn't always like this, hadn't always been like this, wouldn't always be like this. In this moment we made the choice to open to each other, accepting who our partners were, not who we wanted them to be, thought they "should" be. We could see the beauty in them and in ourselves. We couldn't fix the pain or make it go away, but we could love the person through it. And that was all any of us really needed.

Loving Each Other Through Difficult Times: The Story of Sue and George

It's what we long for, really. To be seen, accepted, appreciated, loved. Especially when difficulty has landed squarely on our doorstep, as it did with Sue and George. They found each other later in life, after other heartaches had their way with them. They'd been softened and strengthened by those old heartaches. And they'd been lucky to find love again. Their story, however, didn't end there; it's not " . . . and they lived happily ever after." After they found each other, they each had cancer, and their home burned down. Their life seemed like one hardship after another.

Just when they thought they had rounded the corner, they suddenly found themselves in the midst of a terrifying new health scare, the kind that jolts you into a sudden free fall, disoriented, as if you'd awakened to find the whole world had turned upside down while you were napping. The kind you know could be deadly, though you don't yet know what it actually is. There were trips to the ER, tests, consultations. There was pain and fear, terror even. And time in the ICU with its beeping and buzzing sounds, machines everywhere, wires, monitors, and nurses and doctors responding to the alerts.

Yet in the midst of all this there were moments of certainty, the only certainty that was available to them. One look, one meeting of the eyes, and they knew, without a doubt, that they were loved. Deeply, fully loved. They shared the moment, the pain, the fear, and what held them during this time was their love. They called these moments "green moments" that provided the safety net in this time of life and death. The only safety that Sue and George had. Their only refuge as they navigated this tightrope between life and death.

The Good News: Compassion Can Be Cultivated

You may be reading this and thinking, "That's nice for them, but I'll never feel that. My partner is really challenging to love. Believe me, I've tried." Or "If my partner were different, less demanding, more available, less critical [insert your favorite complaint about your partner here], I could love [him/her/them]. We'd have a much better relationship." Yes, you're probably right. It would be easier if your partner were easier to love.

What I want you to know is that compassion in relationships doesn't depend on your partner. It's a choice. A choice you make, over and over. One you fail to make, then right yourself again and begin anew. Over time the choice becomes a habit and our relationships become safer, more intimate, more satisfying. And that's good news! Compassion can improve our relationships, even if our partner never changes. Truth be told, when we show up with compassion in our relationships, it spills out into the relationships and into our partners. What we bring to the relationship can change the entire course of the relationship. And rather than waiting for our partner to change so compassion can arrive, we ourselves can find it. And that changes everything.

It's also a skill. I used to think that it was just something we were or were not born with. It's true that we are wired differently and some people just have a natural capacity for compassion. Lucky them! And lucky for the rest of us, compassion is a skill that can be cultivated. Like maybe you were a scrawny kid, but you went to the gym and lifted weights and now you're a badass body builder. Sure, there were times when you were injured while trying. So you rested, cared for yourself, asked for help. And then you *tried again*. Each time you failed or were injured you learned something you needed to know, about how to do it in a safer, more effective way. What works, what doesn't. When it matters deeply to you, you keep going, keep showing up.

Failure is just part of the process. It can deepen and strengthen us if we let it. As an LMFT, I'm sometimes asked about how to know if a particular relationship is right for someone. I always inquire about whether they've had difficulties and disagreements yet, and if so, how they were addressed and resolved. We need to know that we can handle difficulties and disappointments together. We need to know that we can count on each other rather than turn on each other. Most of the couples in my psychotherapy practice are working on how to show up in a way that each partner can feel confident they will be met with care and understanding rather than be labeled as the problem. Frankly, what most often brings people in the door is a desire for me to fix their partner. In fact, what actually empowers my patients and helps them to heal their relationships is tending to the places they themselves are wounded and learning how to tend to themselves and each other, rooted in kindness and compassion, rather than letting reactivity run the show.

Our primary relationships are ground zero for reactivity. Even if we are compassionate in most aspects of our lives, it's harder for most of us in our primary relationship. The more important our partners are to us, the deeper our fear of losing them, the more desperate our desire to be loved by them, and the more active our threat/defense system becomes. (We'll explore the threat/defense system in Chapter 2.) We can get into a "can't live with them, can't live without them" quagmire.

Afraid to leave and afraid to get closer. Learning how to strengthen ourselves with compassion gives us both the courage and the motivation to face our fears and tend to ourselves and our relationships in a way that actually makes it safer to be vulnerable with each other, to get closer. To allow ourselves to be known and to be loved. It also gives us the courage to see when our relationship is toxic and we need to leave.

Love Matters

The truth is that we all long to be loved, even if we've shut the door and boarded up the windows to love, all the while shouting "Go away!" out of fear that we'll just be hurt again. There is no getting away from it. Human beings need to belong. We need connection. It's in our wiring. Something in us knows we won't survive alone. From the time we are infants we work to get someone to care about us. We need to be fed and kept warm, to be safe from harm, nurtured, and loved. We cry when we're distressed. Luckily our cries trigger distress in our caregivers too, which cues them to tend to us. Because we are connected, we are wired to pick up, comfort, soothe our babies. And when our babies are content, we are content. When we gaze into their eyes and coo back and forth, our brains and those of our babies are bathed in oxytocin. And that oxytocin actually lays down the gray matter for the capacity to be relational in the future. Connection—good, safe, healthy connection—literally lays the foundation for our capacity to be well connected in our lives.

It's obvious, of course, that without being fed, sheltered, and protected, no baby could survive. What's harder to see is that the connection itself also keeps us alive. When my kids were little, I was friends with another mom, Danae. She had a busy professional life, and she and her husband had been through the difficulties of trying to conceive, without success. After some time they adopted. Their daughter, full of life, was also very physically and emotionally demanding. She never stopped moving or experiencing. The highs were very high and the lows were intense as well. I quite enjoyed being with this little girl, Lisa, but not for too long. She was like a delightful tornado of energy that blew through your house leaving everything off kilter, even if what blew through was a blast of pure sunshine. Her mother was amazing with her. Such patience and kindness, and yet you could feel the toll it took on her, the worn and tired quality of her presence.

Somewhere in the chaos of raising Lisa and maintaining her career, Danae became pregnant naturally, unexpectedly, and her son, Aaron, was born. Aaron was the same age as my middle son, but he was *really* small. As the weeks and months ticked by he didn't grow, and he didn't begin to crawl or walk like our other children. The older my son got, the more he developed, the smaller Aaron seemed. He was no trouble at all, rarely cried or demanded attention of any sort, and yet it was alarming. His parents took him to the pediatrician, who ran many tests. In the end he was diagnosed with failure to thrive. His physical needs were being met reliably, but Aaron had not received enough attention. It's not that Danae and her husband didn't want to tend to Aaron; they did, of course! It's just that they didn't have any energy left over after caring for Lisa. They were moving through the motions of tending to Aaron's needs—changing diapers, feeding him, bathing him—but there was so little of them left that there was no joy and connection in the actions. Aaron needed to be picked up, held, loved, sung to. He needed to belong, to know he was loved. My friends were kind parents, and they loved Aaron, but what he needed most was to be tended to emotionally. He needed to *feel* loved.

And so it is in our primary relationships: we need more than the basics. More than food and shelter, more than who is cooking, taking out the trash, or taking the dog to the vet. We need to *feel loved*. It's the difference between surviving and thriving. Have you drifted into the roles of attending to the basics, and lost touch with feeling loved? It's easy to do in our demanding lives. You're not alone. Or perhaps you are in a space of feeling loved, and you're wise

> In our primary relationships we need more than food, shelter, and other basics—we need to feel loved.

enough to know that it isn't guaranteed. You'd like to do what you can to build the strong foundation that can hold you through the storms of life, sustain you and connect you. Whatever the state of your relationship, we'll explore and develop understanding and practical strategies and exercises that keep your relationship in the healthy zone, or help you find your way back there once again.

The Power of Safe Connection

Beyond our primary relationships we also need connection. In fact, connection has been associated with many health benefits. A study in senior centers found that seniors who had a plant to care for had better health outcomes than those who did not have anything to care for. Several studies have looked at what makes psychotherapy effective and found that the therapeutic alliance between the therapist and patient is a consistent predictor of positive outcomes of treatment. Patients who had a loved one hold their hand when undergoing a painful procedure experienced less pain. What we need most, especially when we are struggling, is each other.

When we have good relationships, we have better outcomes and the painful events of our lives are more tolerable. There is a reason we have rituals that bring us together when we lose a loved one, for example. When the community holds the loss, and the people who are experiencing the loss, the burden is shared. It's like that old teaching story about the woman who lost her son and sought advice on how to bring him back to life. First, she was instructed, you must gather a mustard seed from everyone in the community. As she went door to door collecting the mustard seeds, people asked why she needed the seed, and she explained about her son. Then they shared with her their own stories of loss. After hearing many stories about their losses, she began to understand that loss was a part of life and that she, like them, could survive her loss. In the same way, the more connected we are, the bigger the net beneath us.

I remember when I was in labor with my first child and it wasn't going well. There came a time when my mother kindly looked into my eyes and said, "I wish I could have this baby for you." And she meant it. She wished she could spare me the pain by bearing it herself. It was one of the kindest things anyone has ever said to me. Of course, it didn't change the course of my labor, but it did make it more bearable. Another time I had several health challenges at once, and I didn't understand what was happening to my young and previously healthy body. We didn't have a diagnosis, but my doctor, a fatherly man, gently patted my hand as he reassured me, "We don't know what it is, but we'll figure it out." Everything in me relaxed as I felt seen, tended to, and safe knowing he was on my team and would help me.

There was a particular quality to those relationships. They were characterized by compassion. Compassion notices when we or someone else is suffering, opens to it, recognizes that this is part of our larger shared human condition, holds it with the person suffering, and offers kindness.

Compassion: Kind Connection in Difficult Times

Compassion doesn't look away. It turns toward suffering, offers a kind, connected presence. It's not about fixing our problem or making it go away—though there are certainly times for that. It's about accompanying those on the journey. One of my favorite poets, Naomi Shihab Nye, so beautifully describes compassion in her poem "Kindness," written out of her own experience of traveling through the night on a bus on her honeymoon, when the bus was boarded by bandits. When all was said and done, she found herself in the town square, depending on the kindness of strangers.

> Compassion turns toward suffering; it doesn't look away from it.

Kindness

Before you know what kindness really is
you must lose things,
feel the future dissolve in a moment
like salt in a weakened broth.
What you held in your hand,
what you counted and carefully saved,
all this must go so you know
how desolate the landscape can be
between the regions of kindness.
How you ride and ride
thinking the bus will never stop,

the passengers eating maize and chicken
will stare out the window forever.

Before you learn the tender gravity of kindness,
you must travel where the Indian in a white poncho
lies dead by the side of the road.
You must see how this could be you,
how he too was someone
who journeyed through the night with plans
and the simple breath that kept him alive.

Before you know kindness as the deepest thing inside,
you must know sorrow as the other deepest thing.
You must wake up with sorrow.
You must speak to it till your voice
catches the thread of all sorrows
and you see the size of the cloth.

Then it is only kindness that makes sense anymore,
only kindness that ties your shoes
and sends you out into the day to mail letters and purchase bread,
only kindness that raises its head
from the crowd of the world to say
It is I you have been looking for,
and then goes with you everywhere
like a shadow or a friend.

As Nye observes in her poem, "before you know what kindness really is you must lose things." Compassion doesn't turn away. It opens to, notices, experiences suffering . . . the way you may be experiencing painful feelings about your relationship. It's important not to just power through, not to dull or deaden ourselves, but to allow ourselves to know the truth about our relationship, both the sorrows and the strengths. And this knowing actually opens the door for kindness and compassion to become the "deepest thing inside."

When you open to the truth of your experience of your relationship, what do you see? What are the strengths? The sorrows?

Later in the poem, Nye writes, "you must travel where the Indian in a white poncho lies dead by the side of the road. You must see how this could be you." Here she points to another particular aspect of compassion, shared common humanity. We need to hold our experiences, and those of our loved one, within an understanding of the shared experiences of being human. Being human means that illness, loss, failure, even death, are to be expected for us. There is no way around it. It doesn't mean that there is something wrong with us or our loved one when we struggle in these ways. It doesn't separate us out as uniquely problematic. Not at all, though in our defensive strategies we may want to claim innocence for ourselves as we blame our partner, or criticize ourselves for not feeling loved. That too is human. The truth is that we all struggle and we all behave in ways that are unskillful when we are suffering, to one degree or another. Where did we ever learn that we should be perfect, and our partner too? What a setup! When, with courage, we can see how "this could be me," it softens us, connects us, helps us to recognize that we are all human, no one above or below. We're in this thing together.

Can you see the shared common humanity in your relationship? How your partner also longs to be loved, imperfect as your partner is? How beneath that behavior you don't like is some kind of pain and suffering that your partner has covered over with anger or absence?

Then the poet says, "it is only kindness that makes sense anymore . . . only kindness that raises its head from the crowd of the world to say[,] It is I you have been looking for, and then goes with you everywhere like a shadow or a friend."

The natural result of opening to pain without pushing it away by denying it, blaming it on others, or pretending it couldn't happen to us is kindness. Compassion is simply kindness that is holding pain. And when we learn to hold ourselves

> The natural result of opening to pain without pushing it away is kindness.

and our partner with compassion, we are truly making love, as surely as the alchemist turns lead into gold. We too can use the inevitable pain of life and relationships to make love in our relationships. This is the alchemy of compassion and the secret of good relationships. When we understand our power to transmute our suffering, we develop the habit of turning toward ourselves and our loved ones in times of suffering, rather than turning away. Relationship experts and researchers John and Julie Gottman name this habit of turning toward our partner as one of the core habits that healthy relationships have. Compassion, toward others *and* ourselves, changes the quality of our relationships. In one study, people who were able to extend compassion toward themselves (referred to here as *self-compassion*) were described by their partners as being more emotionally connected, accepting, and "autonomy supporting" and as being less detached, controlling, and verbally or physically aggressive than those lacking in self-compassion. Self-compassion was also associated with greater relationship satisfaction and attachment security. When we can trust each other, even in difficult times, our relationships become characterized by "secure attachment," and that emotional security lays the foundation for our own personal physical and emotional health and for a happy relationship. John Gottman teaches that being friends with our partner is the real secret to a happy relationship.

Beyond the Couple: Well-Connected Relationship Benefits Ripple Outward

And that healthy connection ripples outward. Children in families where parents are securely attached grow up in a healthier environment and are more likely to be securely attached to their caregivers. Sue Johnson, founder of emotionally focused therapy, writes, "When lovers are united in a strong and secure bond, it does more than enhance their connection to each other. The circle of loving responsiveness widens like the ripple from a stone dropped in a pool. Being in a loving relationship augments our caring and compassion for others, in our family and in our community."

The healthy connection in our primary relationship carries beyond our families and into our broader social life, as our presence positively impacts our friendships and forms a base for us beyond our primary relationship. Our net grows broader and deeper, and we find ourselves more courageous and willing to take risks. We can cast our net out in deeper waters and take the risk of living a life that is full and meaningful, whatever that means to each of us.

In that way it also carries into our work lives. Feeling the safe, secure base of a healthy relationship, we can go out into the world and take chances. We can go for that professional goal, trusting that if and when we fail (remember, failure is part of life!), we have a solid net of compassion to fall back on. I think of it as the net under the trapeze. One can take the risk of soaring when there is a soft place to land.

Our own habit of compassion carries into our workplaces too. Google's "Project Aristotle" found that "psychological safety" was by far the most important key dynamic in effective teams. Compassion fosters psychological safety. When we are safely connected with others, our impact in the world increases exponentially. Beyond our workplaces, compassion in our primary relationships sets the foundation for a more compassionate society.

Compassion as a value and a habit in our lives changes all of our relationships. It changes our experience of life itself. And having compassion in our primary relationship ripples outward into the rest of our lives. A compassionate relationship functions like a rudder on a ship, keeping us steady by keeping us in touch with what is deeply meaningful, all the while steering us in the right direction. It offers us strength and vulnerability.

> Compassion as a value and a habit changes our experience of life itself.

Compassion: Strong and Soft

Sometimes people are put off by compassion as they believe it to be soft and fluffy. They think it will make them weak, lazy, and a doormat. This is a common misconception. True compassion has the strength to make hard choices, to set limits, to stand up to harm, to take action. That strength makes it safe to be vulnerable, to open to pain, to feel it, to ask for help, to comfort, soothe, and nurture. It has, as meditation teacher Joan Halifax points out, both a strong back and a soft front. The strong back, like the spine, gives us the strength to be upright, to right ourselves when difficulty tumbles us over, helps us to take a stand for what we value. But it requires a soft front as well. Without that softness the strength becomes brittle and the strong winds can break us. It's the space in the vertebrae that enables the spine to bend rather than break. And, without the soft front, we cannot tolerate the vulnerability of opening to our feelings—so we keep ourselves and our loved ones at a distance when it comes to truly knowing our feelings, and we become isolated from ourselves and our partners.

Just as the strong back requires the soft front, so too does the soft front need the strong back. Without knowing our strength and our capacity to stand up to harm, to set limits, to make hard choices, we may find ourselves blown around by our emotions, completely overwhelmed, unable to take action or even to function.

Compassion has both sides, both faces. And they need each other. Together the strong back and the soft front lead us to wholehearted living, in just the same way that compassion in our primary relationships gives us the courageous vulnerability to develop a more wholehearted life. Fully ourselves.

Healthy relationships need both the strong back and the soft front. What do you most need to cultivate to live fully?

TRY THIS
Finding Strength and Softness

Audio Track 1

Take a moment now to feel into your body:

- Begin by sitting in a comfortable position. Allow your eyes to close if that is comfortable for you. Feel the support of the chair or floor beneath you.

- Knowing you are supported, allow yourself to rest into that support, finding a posture that balances alertness with relaxation, and letting go of any unnecessary tension.

- Bring your attention to your own strong back. Feel how the back supports you and keeps you upright. Even if you have back issues or back pain, still the back is holding you, supporting you.

- Allow yourself to feel your own strength from the inside. If it feels right, you can say to yourself, "Yes, I feel my own strength." Stay here as long as you want.

- Now bring your attention to your soft front. Feel how the

chest and belly gently expand and contract with the movement of the breath in the body. It is this soft front that allows us to be vulnerable, to know our feelings, and to be impacted by the feelings and actions of others. The soft front lets us know the inner and outer world, the way our breathing relates us to the world, taking in what we need and sending out what the trees need.

- Feel the softness, the openness and vulnerability of the front. Know that behind that soft front is a strong back. Stay here as long as you like.

- If you like, feel into the relationship between the strong back and the soft front. Notice how the heart rests in the space between the strong back and the soft front. Feeling the strength of the back, what amount of soft front feels okay now? Feeling the soft front, what amount of strong back feels supportive?

- Take a moment to play with the relationship between the two, knowing that you already have the capacity for both. Are they balanced? Is there an easy flow between the two, or do you find one dominant and the other less familiar?

- Take a moment to notice which one you would like to know better. You can set an intention to notice more of the strong back or more of the soft front as you go about your day.

- Take a moment to notice your wholeness. You have both strength and vulnerability. Thank yourself for showing up and noticing.

Safe Connections: From Surviving to Thriving

Our strength and vulnerability provide the basis for our capacity to be cooperative. Elizabeth Pennisi is a writer for *Science* magazine, with degrees in biology and science writing. Pennisi points out that while

Charles Darwin is often credited with the concept of "survival of the fittest" from his groundbreaking book *On the Origin of Species*; his theory evolved to "survival of the most cooperative" by the time he wrote *The Descent of Man*. Pennisi writes, "The ability to work together provided our early ancestors more food, better protection, and better childcare, which in turn provided reproductive success." And so it is in our relationships—the most cooperative survive. When we work together toward common goals, we are much more likely to achieve them. When we feel safe, we are more likely to be open to connection and cooperation. Compassion is the very thing that provides such safety. Compassionate connection means that when we are at our most vulnerable, we will not be alone. Someone will see us, care about us, and tend to our needs. We are more likely to survive. And beyond survival, we are more likely to thrive.

> Compassionate connection means we won't be alone when at our most vulnerable— we're more likely to survive and even to thrive.

This book is a practical guide to cultivating compassion in our relationships. Having healthy connections makes us more resilient, and that helps us have the courage to go out into the world and accomplish our dreams. Good connection doesn't own us; it empowers us so we can become more fully ourselves. We will explore and build on our capacity to be strong and vulnerable in our relationships. To allow ourselves to be truly, deeply seen. And loved. And to truly, deeply see and love our partners. We can love each other through the ten thousand joys and the ten thousand sorrows of life.

2

"Why Can't You Be Here for Me?"

Understanding What Gets in the Way

It's not the stress that kills us, it is our reaction to it.
—HANS SELYE

Some time ago, when my children were little, I was in the car with one of my friends, Valerie. Valerie was in a really difficult situation. Her husband had an addiction problem so severe that he eventually moved out, was completely overcome by his addiction, and died. At this point he still lived in their home, but his addiction was wreaking havoc within their family. As we were driving, we passed some really fancy homes set on exquisite grounds. We slowed down to look at them. It was dark, and lights glowed inside the houses with their beautifully lit landscaping. I found myself curious about who might live there when I heard Valerie say, "Those people are so happy." "How do you know that?" I asked. "Because just look at their beautiful homes," she said. I laughed and said, "Okay, as long as we're making up stories, that house there has a wife who drinks too much, and in this one over here they're abusing their kids, and the folks in that other one there are in debt up to their eyeballs and can't sleep at night." It is human nature to think that when our conditions improve we'll be happy. But happiness doesn't work like that. We can be surrounded by things our society thinks are blessings, even things we ourselves think are blessings, and we can still be unhappy.

The truth is that life has unavoidable stressors. While a certain amount of wealth and privilege can buffer people from some of the stressors, even many stressors, there is no amount that can shield people from becoming stressed. In fact stress, and the ability to respond to it, is built into our very physiology. This is really important for our survival. Our ancestors who were hanging out in the sun without a care in the world were the ones who got eaten when the predator arrived. There is a protective aspect of stress; it alerts us to danger and gives us the energy to tend to activities that increase the odds of physical survival, like fighting and fleeing. So we need the stress response under certain conditions—mainly ones in which our life is in danger. For that reason, whenever we feel unsafe this system of reactivity becomes the dominant system. The problem is that in our modern world what makes us feel unsafe is usually a threat to our sense of self, our emotional sense of safety, or our sense of being safe in relationship to others, rather than threats to our lives. When the stress response is activated in our relationships, we tend to react in ways that create less safety and more damage in our relationships, rather than more safety. In spite of the harm it causes it's so very common and human.

John and Roberta were an example of this. Married for over thirty years, they had two daughters who were well and truly "launched" and thriving. John was a doctor whose long and fulfilling career had afforded them a beautiful home, relaxing vacations, and a well-funded retirement. Roberta had been a journalist before they had children and then was able to stay home and raise their daughters. In many ways one might say they'd led a blessed life. So why were they in my office for couples therapy? Since John's recent retirement they found themselves vacillating between a cool distance and some really damaging fights in which they each let it be known that their unhappiness rested squarely on the shoulders of the other. And they were each desperate for me to fix . . . their partner.

Far from feeling blessed by their material success and their two daughters, they were very stressed. John felt Roberta's distance and knew she was unhappy with him. He felt like a failure, and he wasn't used to failing, especially at something as important as making his wife happy. He also felt resentful. Hadn't he been a good provider? Hadn't she been able to stay home with their girls and buy whatever she wanted? How dare she make him feel like a failure. He hated feeling like a failure. Sure, he'd tried a few times to give her what she said she wanted, but each time left him feeling worse than before. It seemed he could never get it right in her eyes. So he tended to keep his distance. Work had kept him plenty busy, and then he spent Saturdays golfing. But now that he had retired he had to find new ways to occupy himself. Mostly he felt profoundly lonely, and he was very angry at Roberta for "making him feel that way." They should be having great sex and taking lots of vacations together, he thought. So when she criticized the way he loaded the dishwasher, it was the proverbial straw that broke the camel's back. He exploded in anger and let Roberta know she was impossible to live with, he could never meet her demands, and she never gave him what he needed.

For her part, Roberta already felt like a failure. Why else wouldn't he see her and love her? she wondered. Loneliness was not new to her. Her therapist had once told her that she thought of Roberta as a single mom. While she was raising the girls she was mostly alone. Yes, John had provided them with everything they needed in a material sense, but he was always working when she really needed him. Even when he wasn't working, he was playing golf on Saturdays or watching sports on Sundays. She'd tried to talk with him a few times about how lonely she felt and how overwhelming it was to raise the girls mostly by herself, but John would just tell her he was doing his job supporting the family. He thought perhaps she needed a hobby—how about tennis? When she persisted, he said maybe she needed an antidepressant. She came away feeling even lonelier and more broken. Because she felt like she couldn't count on him for emotional support, her conversations with him centered on the practical details of raising a family and caring for a home. Often her frustration with him was expressed through letting him know how he was not doing things correctly.

In her own way she also became less emotionally available and less vulnerable with him. Being vulnerable seemed only to lead to pain these days. She hardly ever let herself know how deeply she longed for him to notice her and, in some grand romantic gesture, sweep her off her feet. She had waited all these years for him to retire. Work, always the priority, had seemed at times almost like the mistress she couldn't compete with. She told herself that when he retired, she'd finally have his attention, and now he seemed to avoid her. She blamed herself for having settled for so long for someone who didn't seem to value her, and she wondered if she needed to leave him so that she would have a shot at finding someone else and finally feeling loved. And every now and then, after a couple of glasses of wine, she let him know that he was failing her and "he'd ruined her life." She even let him know that she was wondering whether it was wise for her to stay.

The night she told him the dishes needed to be rinsed before they were placed in the dishwasher it all boiled over. She hadn't intended to be critical, but perhaps there had been a tone of frustration in her voice. It was more about not having felt seen and valued when she told him the other fifty times that she really wanted the dishes to be rinsed first. Far from seeing John as incompetent when it came to loading the dishwasher, she saw him as competent. She knew he *could* do it properly, just not if he *would care enough about her* to do it the way she preferred. After all, this had been her domain all these years. She was grateful for the help, but it didn't actually feel like help if she needed to pull the dishes out and rinse them after John loaded the dishwasher. And, she thought, she was really asking for the bare minimum here. Having given up on wanting someone she could feel close with, she was settling for some help with the chores.

John couldn't believe his ears. He'd woken up that morning with the depressed and lonely feeling again. He really longed to be close to Roberta, but when he reached out to hold her she'd gotten out of bed and dressed. He thought maybe, just maybe, if he paid extra attention to doing what she wanted today, she'd warm to him a bit. He folded the clothes and made dinner for her without her noticing. So when she let him know that he wasn't loading the dishwasher right, he just lost it—feeling like she was saying he wasn't worth loving because he didn't load the dishwasher *her way*, like he was just a loser and here was the proof, and like she'd never see him as good and want to get close to him, he launched his counterattack. First, he zeroed in on how actually the *dishwasher* was supposed to wash the dishes, and how ridiculous it was that she wanted him to wash the dishes before putting them in the dishwasher. Roberta felt attacked, so she responded in kind. She wondered, out loud, how he could possibly have run a medical practice without learning how to pick up after himself properly—wounding him in the one place he'd always felt competent. Next, he let her know that she was failing him and that there was indeed something wrong with her in his eyes. He told her she was "a cold fish" and "impossible to please," wondering out loud how anyone could stand to be around her.

Wounded to the core now, Roberta stormed out of the room and into the safety of their bedroom. After locking the door behind her she dove into the bed and lay there sobbing. She didn't want to have anything to do with John. He slept on the couch downstairs that night. In the morning, feeling even worse and knowing that his attack on Roberta had cost him what little closeness they did have, he came to apologize. She let him know how terrible he was, and in an effort to make things safe between them again, he agreed with everything she said as he said he was sorry. Both wondered how they'd gotten here.

John and Roberta's story is more common than you'd think. The tragic part is that both of them long to be seen and loved by the other, yet both have a protective shield up that keeps their partner from being able to safely get close to them. For many of us, that protective shield includes blaming, withdrawing, and placating. Rick Hanson, a psychologist who specializes in cultivating happiness by making positive changes in the brain, talks about our negativity bias. According to Hanson, people tend to be Velcro for negative emotions and Teflon for positive emotions. He notes that we are wired for survival, not for happiness. We are wired to scan our environment for threats! And, according to Barbara Fredrickson, positive emotions expert, when we find a threat our whole world narrows down to just that one problem. This wiring is meant to help us survive. Pausing to notice the beautiful sunset isn't really helpful when a tiger is stalking us. In our lives, however, most of our problems are not life threatening and our physical survival is not at risk. The threat is to our emotional lives, and the way we react often makes the situation worse.

When the Threat/Defense System Kicks In

Psychologist Paul Gilbert, founder of compassion-focused therapy, notes that we have three affect regulation systems—three main ways we manage our emotions. The first is the threat/defense system, the one that John and Roberta were caught in. You may already be familiar with this system. Whenever a threat is present, it is the dominant system in which we automatically find ourselves. It is characterized by reactivity. We don't have to think about how we'll respond; on the contrary, we actually *can't* think. The part of the brain that is responsible for thinking things through and planning (in other words, responding rather than reacting), which is called the *prefrontal cortex*, actually goes offline. We lose access to that part of our brain that would help us reason things through. Instead, powered by the amygdala, our body is dosed with the hormones adrenaline and cortisol as it prepares to protect us by fighting, fleeing, or freezing. We know we are in this system when we feel anger, anxiety, or disgust.

When it comes to relationships, often the threat is to the self. Each of us wants to feel like, and be seen as, a good person. And often what we are fighting off isn't each other . . . it's shame. Our partners may be saying we made a mistake, but it feels like they are saying we *are* a mistake. And because relationships are so important, as we discussed in Chapter 1, especially our primary relationships, it *feels* life threatening when there is a disturbance in the field. So we launch our defensive strategies. Enter the threat/defense system.

> In relationships each of us wants to feel like, and be seen as, a good person. And often what we are fighting off is not each other but shame.

Let's take a closer look at how those protective strategies played out in John and Roberta's case. When Roberta saw the way John was loading the dishwasher without rinsing, she felt unseen, uncared for, and even unsafe emotionally. How the dishwasher was loaded was important to her, and she'd asked him many times in the past to rinse the dishes first. When she saw he wasn't doing it, she experienced a threat to her own well-being and also to the relationship. How could she be safely connected if John didn't see her or care about her? She felt the pain of disconnection, and her threat/defense system was activated. So, although the words she used with John were perfectly kind, the tone she used revealed her irritation. She wasn't really criticizing John; rather she was *protesting the disconnection*. She was in fight mode.

The Fight Mode

John felt the irritation behind the words she used, and feeling the "fight energy" but not understanding where it was coming from, he interpreted it as a threat to his self-worth and their relationship. He assumed she must be thinking he couldn't do anything right and that she didn't think he was worth connecting to. Yikes, that's painful too! Enter John's threat/defense system. He flashed into anger and attacked her by telling her she was "impossible to please" and a "cold fish." His blaming of her was also a sign he was in fight mode. What was really going on for him underneath that anger and blaming was that he was feeling incompetent as a husband and unable to please her. He was desperate for Roberta to like him so that he could feel he was worth something. After all, the one area where he had felt compe-tent—work—was no longer available to him. So when he lashed out at Roberta and blamed her for his feelings, he was just trying to protect his image of himself as a good person who was worthy of love. He was trying to fend off the shame of feeling like he was a bad person for dis-appointing her. It wasn't really about Roberta herself; she'd just pushed the button. In the same way, it wasn't really about John's competence when she complained that he wasn't loading the dishwasher properly. That had really been about her longing to feel seen, heard, valued, and loved. They had each made the mistake of thinking the other person's behavior was about them. And they each reacted to the threat in ways that created a downward negative spiral in their relationship.

The Flight Mode

When John lashed out at Roberta, what he said wounded her to the core. Instinctively, she understood that if she continued to stay and fight with John she would be further wounded and that she couldn't take much more. So she moved into flight mode. She stormed out and sought safety in her bedroom. Withdrawal is another strategy

Sometimes we withdraw to protect ourselves and sometimes to protect the relationship.

for self-protection. We do this sometimes to protect ourselves and sometimes to protect the relationship. We know that continuing to engage in fighting is causing harm to the relationship, so we choose to withdraw in an effort to protect it. This can be an important strategy that allows the activation from the threat/defense system to settle, but when it is done in a way that feels like abandonment to the other person, it adds fuel to the fire and stokes the threat/defense system even further. The other person now feels desperate to connect, as John did, locked out of the bedroom and unable to connect with Roberta.

The Freeze Mode

John's threat/defense system was on red alert. It felt like a death spiral. Because he was unable to fight or flee his way out of the situation, the final threat/defense mode kicked in—placating. In an effort to preserve the connection with Roberta, he set out to please her. Well, not please her exactly, more like placate her. If he could remove the sense of threat she was feeling, then maybe they could connect again. This wasn't a thought-out process; it was characterized by the reactivity of the threat/defense system. He found himself agreeing with everything she said and apologizing. If he agreed with her about everything, she'd settle down. The problem was that he didn't actually agree with everything she said. For example, he didn't agree that the dishes needed to be rinsed first. He thought he knew better than she did, which was why he didn't follow through on his past promises to rinse the dishes first. He didn't even really remember those conversations because he wasn't really present. He didn't show up, vulnerability and all, and take the risk that it would feel worse before they eventually managed to work things out. He also didn't agree with Roberta's assessment that he didn't care about her. In fact, she was the most important person in the world to him. But in placating her he apologized for not caring enough about her. And in this way he let Roberta's underlying story about not being important to John and loved by John grow stronger. Roberta could sense that this apology was designed to make her calmer, rather than truly address the pain she was feeling, which only heightened her sense of feeling unseen and unloved.

Can you see the physiology of the threat/defense system at play here? The threat/defense system is characterized by fight/flight/freeze. The system is activated when we feel threatened, so the main goal of the system is protection and safety seeking. We want to be safe. It's our hardwired survival instinct in play here. Think about it for a moment: if you were on the battlefield, there would be three main strategies you could deploy. First, you could fight and defeat your opponent. That would protect you from the threat. A second strategy would be to flee. If you could outrun your opponent, you could also protect yourself and get to safety. If neither of those strategies seemed possible, then as a last resort you might freeze, play dead. It would seem like you were no longer a threat to your opponent, and your opponent might move on and pass you by, which could also restore safety for you. This threat/defense system is lifesaving. If you find yourself on the battlefield, this is *the* system you need. So it's not a bad system at all. It just doesn't work so well when we use it to battle our partners.

Exploring Your Own Style

Many couples, like John and Roberta, find themselves in the threat/defense system frequently. Your own situation might not look exactly like theirs. We all have our preferred defense mechanisms. Some relationships are characterized by explosive fights, like John and Roberta's, while others are characterized by what my colleague Chris Germer refers to as the "cold hell"—lots of distance and not much warmth. Here, both people are withdrawn. Other situations may be characterized by a surface friendliness and warmth but a lack of true connection, leading to a

> Hiding ourselves from each other keeps us from feeling seen and loved.

sense of deep loneliness and confusion since things appear warm on the surface. These relationships are characterized by placating, an effort to preserve the relationship by not making waves. When we hide ourselves from each other, we can't feel seen and loved.

When the threat/defense system is active in our relationships, we may find ourselves engaging in some of these behaviors:

Fight: criticize, argue, deny, defend, scowl, roll the eyes, blame

Flight: storm out of the room, sneak away, pretend not to hear, withdraw our presence

Freeze: apologize profusely, agree with everything our partners say, placate

Typically, each of us will have developed a primary strategy for our threat/defense system, based on our past experiences. We may be willing to fight if we think we can win. If we don't think so, or we think it would be too damaging, we may try to withdraw. If neither of those options seems possible, freeze becomes our default strategy. It is actually characterized by surrender out of an inability to do anything. The body is both on red alert and immobilized. And these become habitual, so that how we behave tends to be based on our past behaviors and experiences. Yes, there are situational influences too. When our primary patterns aren't available to us, we often go to the other strategies.

Since these strategies are habitual and have likely become automatic, it is helpful to know what each of these states feels like so you have a better chance of recognizing when you are in them. Here are some ways people feel in the threat/defense system. You may feel differently. The point is to become familiar with your own cues that you are in the threat/defense system.

Fight: hot face, heart racing, muscles tense, raised voice

Flight: antsy, energy in the legs, can't hear, withdrawing

Freeze: walking on eggshells, holding breath, confused, surrendering

TRY THIS
Uncovering Your Survival Strategies

Audio Track 2

Take a moment to think of a time when you were having a disagreement with your partner.

Remember, if you can, how the problem started. Then replay the situation in your mind, step by step, as if you were replaying a video of the incident in slow motion.

Use the pause button to remember the feelings you were having and identify which strategies you used.

Each of these defense strategies has a particular feel to it.

You might pause for a moment and see what happens in your body as you remember being in each of these states. Notice what it feels like in *your body* when you are in fight mode, flight mode, or freeze mode. This will help you recognize when you're in each mode in the future.

See if you can drop underneath the defensive strategies now and feel into what softer, more vulnerable feeling lies below them. What were you *really* trying to protect yourself from? Were you fighting off feeling like a bad person (shame)? Feeling unlovable? Feeling lonely? Feeling unseen? See what it is for you. Is this a familiar feeling?

Now imagine you had a friend who was feeling this way. What would you say to your friend?

Try offering yourself the same message. Perhaps something like "I'm here for you" or "I see you" or "You matter to me, and I'll be there for you." See what it is for you and offer yourself your own kindness.

If you can, you might also receive your own kind words. Let them in.

How do you feel right now? You might make a note to yourself about:

- Which strategies you used
- What it felt like in your body with each strategy

- What that strategy was protecting you from (the softer feeling underneath)
- What you needed (what was helpful to be reminded of with your words)

You can use these notes to help you become more aware of what you really need when you find yourself in threat/defense mode.

Could you see that underneath the defensive strategy was pain? Could you identify the wounded person there? Beneath your protective strategies is a person who is suffering. At any given moment when our suffering exceeds our resources, bad or unskillful behavior is the likely result. It's human nature. And that doesn't make us bad, though our actions may really harm others. It makes us human. We all behave in ways that are harmful at times. It may not make us bad, but it does create harm. Let's explore that more deeply now.

TRY THIS

How Your Survival Strategies Affect Your Partner

Audio Track 2

Imagine you were on the other side of the defensive behavior you identified in the preceding exercise. Your partner blamed you, left you, or reflexively apologized to you, for example.

See if you can feel what it would be like to be on the receiving end of this behavior.

- What feelings do you have?
- What does it feel like in your body?
- Do you want to get closer to your partner?
- Are you willing to be vulnerable?

Can you see the harm the defensive behavior causes to your partner and your relationship? Can you see how it gets in the way of achieving the kind of relationship you want? Again, it's helpful to remember that we are wired this way. These are common

> When our suffering exceeds our resources, the result is likely to be bad or unskillful behavior.

behaviors, and you are certainly not alone! We are wired for survival, not for happiness. And unless your life is actually in danger, which sadly is sometimes the case, this isn't the best system for you to use when you are in conflict with your partner. I did also point out that it is automatic, so where's the hope here?

The answer is that this system kicks in when we feel threatened, and it is designed to restore safety. When it comes to relational threats, there are much better ways to restore safety. Accordingly, we have a responsibility to ourselves and our loved ones to build the skills that increase our resources so that we can create the conditions for safety in our relationships and develop healthier, kinder relationships. Ones that are characterized by safe, connected presence, as we'll explore further as the book unfolds.

Our Partners Are Human Too

While we are on the topic of looking at how our own bad or unskillful behavior has its roots in our own pain and in feeling threatened, we have an opportunity to see that the same is true for our partners. When they behave in ways that are unskillful and hurt us, we need to keep in mind that their behavior is really a reflection on *them*. And far from saying that it's because they are bad, what it actually says is that they are in pain right now. This doesn't mean we have to tolerate bad behavior. In fact, each of us also has a responsibility not to participate in harm, which may mean setting a strong limit with your partner. (If your partner's behavior *is* life threatening for you, the threat/defense system may be a better choice; in the United States, the National Domestic Violence Hotline number is 800-799-7233.)

It doesn't mean you have to tolerate your partner's bad behavior, but it does mean that you make a mistake when you take the behavior personally. The behavior wasn't about you, even if your partner says it was. Really the behavior is a reflection on their own pain. It speaks volumes about how *they are feeling* right now. If John had been able to pause when he felt criticized and see that it wasn't about him or how he loaded the dishwasher, things would have been different. If he could have felt that extra energy in Roberta's comment and seen that as a cue that *she was in distress,* he would have had an opportunity to be curious with her about her distress. That would have sent an entirely different message to her. Instead of feeling unseen, she would have felt seen and cared about, and an upward, healing relational pattern would have begun. If Roberta could have seen John's insults as a clue that *he was suffering,* she could have let him know that insulting her wasn't helpful and been curious with him about his distress— again, creating an upward relational spiral. Kindness begets kindness. Understanding that your partner's unskillful behavior is a clue that *your partner* is suffering, rather than taking the behavior personally, changes everything. And it can be the start of developing a better relational pattern.

3

"I Wish I Could Fix It!"
Resisting Pain with Problem Solving

> Don't meditate to fix yourself, to heal yourself, to improve
> yourself, to redeem yourself, rather, do it as an act of love,
> of deep warm friendship to yourself.
> —BOB SHARPLES

In my work with couples and families I often talk about how we "catch the flu" from each other. What I mean by that is when one person gets angry, the other often gets angry too. Or when one thinks something is funny, the other often catches the feeling. Scientists have a name for this: emotion contagion. Emotion contagion has its roots in the mirror neuron system, a network in the brain that helps us understand others and forms the basis for empathy.

One particular memory arises when I think about emotion contagion. It was a long time ago. My oldest was just a toddler, and his brother would have been about three months old. They were so close in age that I had a twin stroller, with them facing each other. The toddler had a condition that required him to wear prescription shoes. We had just come from the shoe store, and they gave us a helium balloon, which we had tied to the stroller. The oldest was tugging on the ribbon that tethered the balloon to the stroller, and the balloon was bouncing up and down. The baby started to belly laugh. It's quite something when a baby that small is belly laughing. Then the toddler began to laugh. Then I caught the laughter, along with my husband. And there we were, the four of us walking through the shopping mall, laughing hysterically over . . . nothing at all, actually. I didn't find the bouncing balloon to be funny. But I'd caught the laughter from my children, and now we couldn't stop. Tears ran down my cheeks. My belly and cheeks hurt from laughing so hard. My laughter was reinforcing theirs, and theirs was reinforcing mine. It's a pleasant memory for me.

Unfortunately, we also catch undesirable emotions from each other. Have you ever gotten angry at someone who is angry at you, or felt overwhelming sadness when you're with someone who has just experienced a loss? Like it or not, we feel others' feelings too. Often, we can easily understand and empathize with the person having those feelings. This ability to feel others' emotions, called empathic resonance, is important, as it forms the basis for compassion. But empathy without the buffer of feelings of love (which arise in the care system, as we'll explore later) just has us marinating in pain and can feel unbearable. The person whose pain it is may not have a choice in the situation. Loss is painful, for example; there is no way around that. Yet, because we catch emotions from each other, being around people who are sad (or angry, or frightened, etc.) may make us feel sad (or angry, or frightened, etc.)—and most of us would prefer to avoid situations that increase our own undesirable emotions.

If we can't tolerate the feelings they (and we) are having, we can move into strategies to get them to stop having that undesired emotion around us—we might try to make them stop by shaming or blaming them. In other words we are *resisting* opening to things as they are and to our partners as they are. Or we may be tempted to spend less time with them—avoid them so we avoid having our own undesired feelings triggered—another form of *resisting* being with our partners as they are. But we don't want to abandon our loved ones when they need us. After all, we want to be with *them*—just not their painful emotions. We develop strategies to get them out of the pain they are in so we can be with them without feeling their pain. This activates another of our three affect regulation systems: the drive system.

The Drive System

The drive system is another emotion regulation system Paul Gilbert describes. It helps us access resources we need. We need things like food, clothing, and shelter, and it is the drive system that we engage to help us gather resources and solve problems. When we achieve our goals of solving a problem or getting something that we need or want, we are "rewarded" with a hit of dopamine. Dopamine is the pleasure hormone and neurotransmitter. It feels good to solve our problems and to gather resources. Like the threat/defense system, the drive system is a good system to have and to engage. It is also an activating system. The sympathetic nervous system is activated, which functions like the gas pedal in a car. It gives us the energy to get what we need. We do need to solve problems and access resources; that's part of keeping ourselves alive. The problem comes when we use the drive system in an attempt to get out of *emotional* pain.

The drive system doesn't do a good job of helping us avoid emotional pain. Of course, there are times when we do need to seek the resources that will allow us to solve our problems. However, when we are in emotional pain, what we usually need first is to not be in pain alone. We seek the comfort of "safe others." We need others to hold us while we are experiencing pain. When we let someone know we are having a hard time, it feels terrible when the person doesn't acknowledge our pain and instead just tells us how to solve our problem— or how *they think* we could solve our problem. We feel unseen and unloved. And eventually, if others have felt unsafe for us, we may find we prefer not to be with anyone else and risk adding relational pain to our already existing emotional pain.

When the drive system is functioning well in relationships, it helps us do things like buy a home, raise a family, and plan a vacation. The drive system can be really satisfying relationally. It helps us to do things together, as a team, and to accomplish shared goals. However, we often use the drive system to avoid feeling someone else's emotional pain, and that never turns out well for us. In relationships there are at least three main ways we behave when we engage the drive system to resist pain: fixing, controlling, and criticizing. Let's look at each of these in more detail.

> We often use the drive system to avoid feeling someone else's emotional pain, which never works out well.

Strategy 1: Fixing

One of our go-to strategies is fixing. Fixing has its roots in good intentions. If we can help rid the other person of pain, everyone will feel better. What could be wrong with that? The problem is that fixing also has its roots in resistance. One definition of resistance I like is "wishing things were other than they are." When we push away the reality of what is, we also unintentionally dismiss the person who is experiencing that reality. Despite our good intentions, fixing usually makes the situation worse, not better.

Monica and Jason were caught in this dilemma. Monica was having a terrible time at work. When she was growing up, her mother cleaned houses and her father worked as a handyman. Her parents worked hard, and the family always had enough, but sometimes it felt like barely enough. Monica was smart, and because of her parents' hard work she was able to go to a decent school and focus on her schoolwork. Her teacher, Ms. Faust, noticed she was smart and willing to work hard, and she encouraged Monica to go to college. Monica was proud to be the first in her family to get a college degree. Although she had many challenges along the way, Monica did really well in her professional career. She did so well that when their kids came along, Jason was able to stay home with the kids while Monica supported the family. Jason was really proud of Monica's success, and he loved being able to be home with the kids.

Then Monica's company changed its structure. The department she ran was moved into another group where she reported to a new boss, Stacey. That's when the trouble began. No matter what Monica did, she never seemed able to please Stacey. That was two years ago. Monica was miserable!

Jason was really concerned. Monica used to come home happy, even after working long hours. He would listen as she described her projects at work. He loved seeing the joy and satisfaction on her face as she recounted her day. Even if he'd had a hard day himself, he found himself smiling and taking pleasure in her success. It reminded him of life beyond diapers and dishes. But for the past two years, he had been watching Monica grow more and more discouraged and depressed. Now she didn't want to talk about work, except every now and then when she'd break down in tears about how demoralizing it all was and how she felt. She felt trapped by Stacey. And in a larger sense, she felt trapped by being the sole provider for her family. She felt pressure to maintain their lifestyle. Jason could feel her slipping away, and that scared him.

Monica was scared too. She was scared that she seemed unable to avoid letting everyone down. The longer it went on, the more broken-spirited she became and the less able she actually was to get her job done. She found herself checking out at work and felt terribly guilty about it. She was tired all the time and didn't seem to enjoy life anymore. She even found herself eating more junk food and gaining weight.

The more withdrawn Monica became, the more Jason tried to fix her. When she complained about her weight gain, he told her she needed to try the keto diet. When she complained about being tired all the time, he told her she needed to see the doctor and have a physical. He thought maybe her thyroid was out of balance. When she complained about not enjoying life, which was only once or twice, he told her she was depressed and needed to see a psychiatrist. Ouch, that one really hurt! She had come away feeling like she was crazy on top of everything else. And when she complained about her boss, he told her she needed to get a new job. How, she thought, can I do that when I'm already barely keeping up with everything? Jason always seemed to have solutions, but none of them actually felt helpful to Monica.

Jason was getting really tired of listening to the same problems over and over and was growing more desperate for Monica to do something about them. He could feel her pain, and it felt overwhelming and scary. She had been his rock. Deep down, in ways he wasn't conscious of, he was feeling really vulnerable. What would happen if Monica didn't take care of her health and he lost her? That was a grief he didn't want to imagine or endure. And what would happen if Monica lost her job or quit? He'd also grown up in a home that had struggled to make ends meet, and he didn't want to experience that again. Nor did he want to be back in the job market himself and face the threat that *he* would be in a difficult environment. So, without even being aware of his own vulnerability and fears, he found he couldn't help telling Monica how she should solve her problems. For most of us, it is easier to focus on others' problems, so we don't have to focus on our own.

For Monica, his advice just felt like more to do and more reminders that she was a failure. What she really needed, she told Jason, was just for him to listen to her and let her know that he loved her. She just wanted him to sit in the vulnerability with her and love her through this challenging time. When Jason tried to fix her, she felt like she was a burden or a problem to be solved. She felt unseen and unloved, and it left her rather hopeless. She *wanted* to feel that she was loved and that whatever happened she wouldn't have to face it alone. And, yes, she would also like to have the problems solved.

> What we often need is for our partners to sit in our vulnerability with us and love us through those challenging times.

Maybe you're reading this and thinking that you can relate! If so, which side do you land in? Maybe, like Jason, you identify with the frustration of knowing you could solve the problem, if only your partner would listen and take your advice. Then you wouldn't have to keep hearing about how it hurts. You're tired of feeling your partner's pain and know there is a simple and effective solution available to get out of that pain. Maybe you aren't even aware that underneath your solutions you're feeling more vulnerable than you would like.

Or maybe you identify more with Monica. You're trying to describe the hard time you are having, and your partner keeps trying to tell you how to fix it. Although you can see that you do have a problem and you would eventually like to solve it, you just wish your partner would listen. You don't need your partner to solve the problem; you simply want them to care that you're having a problem and to hold that problem with you.

Whichever side you identify with, I bet you can feel the frustration and stuckness. If only your partner would do it differently, things would be better. If only she would get a new job. If only he would listen.

What's going on here?

This scenario has its roots in the threat/defense system. Monica is clearly feeling depressed, demoralized, and hopeless. We feel each other's pain, especially the pain of those we are closest to. So, she isn't the only one in pain here. Jason is also in pain. It's hard to see Monica struggling at work. And it's even harder to listen to her describe how painful it is and all of the problems it is causing. He is feeling *her pain* and he is also feeling *his own vulnerability.* He doesn't want her to be in pain, and he doesn't want to be vulnerable to things that would cause him more pain either. So he tries to *fix her pain and make it go away.* I call it the circuitous route. Rather than tending to his own pain so he can stay with her, he attempts to fix the root of the pain by fixing her. If he can do that, they'll both be pain free. A good solution, it seems. After all, life was good before this job change—and it could be again!

But Monica is having none of it. In fact, he is irritating her! So now, in addition to the problems caused by her work and health, there is this added layer of frustration with Jason—relational pain on top of everything else. Getting a new job and a physical may indeed be what she needs on a practical level, but she first wants to be tended to relationally. Then she'll likely be open to solutions for her job situation and physical health.

Another way to look at it would be that she is feeling vulnerable and is swimming in feelings. Remember the strong back/soft front from Chapter 1? She's squarely in the soft front—in touch with her vulnerability, feeling her feelings, and looking to the relationship for comfort and soothing. She is seeking Jason's strong back to *help her hold the pain*, so she needs him also to be able to open to vulnerability. Jason, however, would prefer to *skip over* the pain and vulnerability of the soft front and get right to the strong back. He wants to take action and solve the problem without also being in touch with the soft front. This leaves Monica feeling abandoned.

Neither of them is wrong! That's really important to recognize. Whichever position you identify with, you aren't wrong. And neither is your partner. Both things need to happen. The answer lies in the order in which we proceed. In this case, Monica first needs to be seen and validated. She needs to feel Jason's loving, connected presence. Her soft front needs his soft front first. If he can meet her there, the physiology of her threat/defense system will settle. Once she feels calm, connected, and safer, her prefrontal cortex will come back online and she'll be better able to solve the problem. She may even welcome

Jason's input and strong back then. It turns out this is a common pattern for most of us. When we inevitably find ourselves in the threat/defense system, we move into the drive system. It's our attempt at a strong back, but without a simultaneous soft front, it becomes fixing.

First Offer Your Kind, Connected, Presence

As we've already noted, Monica and Jason's situation illustrates what it looks like when we engage in fixing. We can see that the fixing strategy doesn't work when Jason deploys it. No one wants to feel like a problem to be solved or a burden to be endured. No one wants to feel like they need to be fixed before they can belong. As Bob Sharples goes on to explain in the quote at the top of this chapter, there is "the subtle aggression of self-improvement." Partner improvement can also feel like subtle (or not so subtle) aggression. When we are struggling and turn to others for support, we are looking for a response that is grounded in their kind presence, with a sense of understanding based in our shared human condition. We seek acknowledgment that it's normal to feel this way and we are not alone.

> When we are struggling, we seek support from others—understanding of our shared human condition and acknowledgment that it's normal to feel this way.

Don't take my word for it. See what happens for you as you try the following exercise.

TRY THIS

Discovering What Is and Isn't Helpful When We Have Problems

Think about a time when you went to your partner or a friend because you had a problem and you wanted support, but you were offered solutions.

How did that feel for you?

What did you need from this person?

As in Monica's case, you probably just wanted the person to listen. When someone listens to us, offering us their loving, connected presence, we begin to feel safer, cared about, and connected. We feel accepted and acceptable just as we are. We stop feeling like we are all alone in this, and that sense of affiliation and belonging begins to calm our physiology. When we are struggling and turn to someone for support, we are usually looking for three things, whether we know it or not: mindfulness, common humanity, and kindness. We need someone to be with us as we are. In other words, we need the other person's presence. That's the mindfulness part. We also need a sense that we are connected and that the others we need to listen to us don't see themselves as better than us. Rather, they can relate to us. They know our situation could happen to them too. They see the shared human condition. That's the common humanity part. The natural result of opening to our pain and feeling connected is caring. Their caring feels like love. That's the kindness part.

> When we turn to someone for support at a difficult time, we are usually looking for mindfulness, common humanity, and kindness.

It sounds easy, doesn't it? When we train our minds and hearts in compassion, it can be. Yet that's not where most of us start. It isn't just others that get into fixing mode. It's human nature. We all do it. Let's explore our own tendency to fix.

TRY THIS

Discovering Our Tendencies to Fix

Audio Track 3

Think about a time when someone you cared about was in distress and you felt the person's distress. Perhaps you felt their distress so much it felt nearly unbearable.

Did you offer them solutions? Tell them how you solved a similar problem or what they need to do to solve their problem?

What effect did it have on them?

Can you see that in spite of your good intentions, it may have felt bad for this person you care about?

It's likely, as in Jason's case, that helping a loved one solve their problem felt like an act of love for you. You may have felt overwhelmed by their pain. And you wanted to stop seeing your loved one in pain. You wanted to have some control in the painful situation, and you tried to help in a way that would stop the pain, both yours and theirs. If so, you also know what it feels like to engage the drive system by way of fixing in order to avoid pain. How did it work out for you? Did the other person appreciate your trying to fix them?

Now that you have explored what it feels like on both sides of fixing, perhaps you're noticing that even if there are good intentions underneath, fixing as a way of getting out of pain usually just increases pain.

Strategy 2: Controlling

I mentioned above that fixing can have its roots in wanting to have some control in the situation. In fact, controlling is another of the strategies we often deploy in an effort to avoid pain. Many times this strategy is deployed in a preventive way. There is a delusion that if we and our loved ones just do everything right, we can prevent bad things from happening. There is a fantasy of omnipotence in there. We may wish to be that powerful, but truly we are not. Bad things happen anyway, even when we try hard to do everything right. Should we try to do things that better our chances of being successful? Absolutely! And we also have to be mindful of our attachment to outcome. When we know that we aren't 100 percent in control of that outcome and we show up anyway, we are in the healthier part of the drive system. When we frantically and obsessively try to control the situation so that *we avoid pain*, we have veered into the unhealthy use of the drive system, and our efforts are likely to cause more problems.

Take the case of Katie and Sarah. Katie grew up in the Midwest with an alcoholic father. In her early years, she remembers being close to her father as they worked on cars together. Later in her childhood, however, his drinking became a problem. When he drank, he became mean. Katie and her sisters could hear the way he verbally and some-times physically abused their mother when he was drunk. And it didn't stop there. He also became emotionally abusive to them. He was scary, and they were terrified. Eventually, Katie's mother took the girls to a domestic violence shelter, and together they started over without their father. They moved to California and began new lives.

Some time later, on a visit back to the Midwest to see her relatives, Katie met Sarah. She loved Sarah's sense of playfulness and her sense of humor and adventure. Sarah was full of life, and it felt like a breath of fresh air to Katie. Sarah loved Katie's reliability and the way she seemed to know just what to do at all times. She felt like she could really count on Katie to be present and to care about her. Sarah breathed life, fun, pleasure, and a sense of aliveness back into Katie's life, and Katie brought security and stability back into Sarah's life. They fell deeply in love. It was a long-distance relationship, and they traveled frequently to spend time at each other's homes. It felt like a dream come true, and they began to explore how they might combine their households into one.

But along the way, Katie began to notice Sarah's drinking. Katie had sworn off alcohol altogether since it had caused so much harm in her family of origin. She was, frankly, uncomfortable being around people who drank. She tried to keep an open mind. She knew that not all people who had a glass of wine had a drinking problem. Still, just seeing the glass of wine set off alarm bells in her. She found herself paying really close attention to Sarah's drinking. She noticed how full the glass was, for example. Wasn't that an overpour? she wondered. What Sarah counted as one serving seemed more like two to Katie. And when Sarah poured herself a second drink, Katie registered that as four glasses, and her system was now on red alert. When she brought up the topic with Sarah, there was a bit of a charge to it. She let Sarah know that her pours were too heavy. She let her know that she was actually consuming four glasses of wine and that wasn't okay. Katie didn't intend to be insulting. She was scared. Sarah was so important to her, and she was scared of losing Sarah—and even more frightened of becoming unsafe again. So she scrutinized what Sarah consumed and tried to control it.

Sarah couldn't believe what she was hearing. She usually could count on feeling loved and supported by Katie, and now Katie didn't seem to believe in her. Katie felt the need to monitor every drop of wine Sarah drank, and Sarah frankly found that insulting. Didn't

Katie trust her anymore? Suddenly she felt more like Katie was the enemy, just waiting to catch how bad she was. Sarah felt diminished by Katie's controlling behavior. It was hard for her to see that Katie's controlling behavior was rooted in her love for Sarah and in Katie's own fears from the past. If Sarah had truly seen that, she might have been willing to limit her drinking, not to please Katie or get her off her back, but out of a sense of love and care for Katie. In this case, Katie's effort to control Sarah led to a downward spiral of distrust. Katie didn't trust Sarah to manage her alcohol, and Sarah, feeling the distrust, didn't trust that Katie was on her side and had her best interests at heart. Things devolved from there.

The more deeply someone or something matters to us, the more likely it is that control will surface as a strategy to ensure safety. This often happens in relationships where one person has very high standards for housework or childcare, for example. Sometimes the standards are so high that it's difficult for a partner to meet them. The partner, feeling frequently corrected or criticized for failing to live up to the standards, often fears failure, and at some point disengages from attempts to live up to the expectations and avoids responsibility in these areas. As that partner does less in an attempt to avoid chronic failure, the high-standards partner does more. Whenever one partner overfunctions, the other partner is likely to underfunction. The overfunctioning partner not only risks burnout and frustration but is also likely to feel unloved when left to do all of the work. It is hard for the overfunctioner to see that his partner's underfunctioning isn't actually about love. It's about wanting to be free from control and fearing failure.

When we use control as a strategy to prevent bad things from happening, we skip over the other person. No one wants to feel controlled. And no one wants to fail their partner. Both are painful outcomes of a strategy intended to prevent pain.

TRY THIS

Discovering What's Underneath the Need to Control

Audio Track 4

Think about a time when you wanted your partner to change a behavior.

How did you communicate your desire that your partner change? Was there a bit of a charge to it or perhaps an edge in your tone? Could your partner have felt criticized?

If so, see if you can dive under the desire for the behavior change and identify your underlying fear or vulnerability. What were you afraid would happen if your partner didn't change?

You may have to continue asking yourself the question and diving under the layers of fear to see the true vulnerability you were trying to avoid.

This isn't an easy exercise, is it? It's hard to really see our core vulnerabilities. When we do, we can simply reassure ourselves, just like we would a dear friend, that having that fear makes sense. We can reassure ourselves, too, that we'll tend to our needs as best we can, even (and especially) when our partner lets us down. In the next chapter, we'll explore how to tend to ourselves and each other more fully. For now, it is enough to see how our efforts to avoid our vulnerability can feel like criticism to our partners.

TRY THIS

What Your Partner Feels When You Try to Control

Audio Track 4

Now imagine you were on the other side of that criticism.

What would it feel like to receive the message with that charged tone?

Even if you could see that you *were* failing in some way, what would you wish for from your partner?

What we really want is to be seen and accepted as we are. We want to know that, in spite of our shortcomings, we also have good qualities and overall we are lovable. When we feel lovable and we understand the vulnerability of our partners, we are often motivated to make changes out of love rather than fear or resentment. As the renowned psychologist Carl Rogers put it, "The curious paradox is that when I accept myself as I am, then I can change." Our partners can too.

TRY THIS

Speaking from Vulnerability

Audio Track 4

Now, in touch with your own vulnerability and that of your partner, is there a way that you could address the situation differently if you find it still needs to change?

What if you practiced by freely and spontaneously writing a letter to your partner?

This letter is just for you—you don't need to give it to your partner.

I've seen, many times, people attempt to prevent bad things from happening by doing everything right. I have never once seen it result in no bad things happening, but I have often seen it result in burnout and relational pain. What works much better than trying to exert control is resting in our resilience. When we know that we have the capacity to care for ourselves and each other when things go poorly, our physiology relaxes a bit. The prefrontal cortex (and our ability to think things through) comes back online, and together we can find our way to respond to the problem, like Sue and George from Chapter 1, who managed to have their "green moments" in the midst of fear and pain over a major health crisis. They didn't simply rest in their loving connection. Rather, their loving connection provided the support they needed to endure the challenging process of medical recovery.

Strategy 3: Criticizing

The third thing I often see people do when they are in their drive system trying to get out of pain is criticize. Even if you don't think you are criticizing, your partner may *feel* criticized. John and Roberta in Chapter 2 are a good example. Roberta didn't intend to criticize John for the way he loaded the dishwasher. She was really just trying to improve his dishwashing skills. It was important to her that the dishes got washed well. At least that was how it began for her. For Roberta, keeping the house clean and organized makes her feel safer. It is her way of preventing bad things from happening. So her requests about loading the dishwasher correctly are really requests that John keep her safe by helping her feel in control of her environment. When John repeatedly failed to load the dishwasher correctly, Roberta felt unsafe, unheard, and unloved. Thus her requests became more and more charged with urgency and the pain of feeling unloved.

The message John heard was "You're not doing it well." At best, he heard "You need to improve." At worst, he heard "You're such a failure, you can't even load the dishwasher properly. You're useless." And the more Roberta repeated the message to John, the more he got the harshest message instead of the milder one. John had no idea that Roberta's energy was more about her pain than it was about his performance. For that matter, it was largely an unconscious process for Roberta too.

In these situations, we may feel like we're just trying to improve our partners. We often don't realize that we're also trying to avoid pain. We feel we are making suggestions from a place of love. When it is truly just out of love, however, our partners don't usually feel criticized by our comments. When there is a bit of a charge to the comments or a bit of an edge in our tone, our partners pick up on it, and that extra energy gets interpreted as criticism. That extra energy is often some sort of fear sneaking in—fear you may not even be aware of.

Maybe your partner has a big presentation to give at work and you notice that his outfit isn't exactly flattering. What do you do? You want others to see the best of him. You want your partner to be successful. Should you say something? What do you say? If you say, "That isn't your best look; why don't you try the blue pants?" your partner may come away feeling criticized and undermined. Instead of feeling confident, he now feels a little less confident. Even if you are coming mostly from a good place, it's likely that if you have a bit of a charge when you speak with him, your partner will come away feeling criticized. When your partner feels criticized, he shuts down a bit. Of course, sometimes the criticism is markedly sharp and pointed. This profoundly undermines us and shuts us down. It is worth mentioning here that we are often really harsh with ourselves. Whether it is self-criticism or partner criticism, feeling like a failure often has the effect of demotivating us.

What we really long for is to be seen and accepted just as we are. Why can't our partners do that for us? Why can't we do that for our partners? In the example above, you might notice that your partner's outfit isn't the most flattering, and you're aware of wanting him to look his best. What you probably aren't aware of is your own fear of what will happen if he doesn't. Maybe you worry that he'll reflect poorly on you. What would people think of you for being with a partner so unattractive? Or maybe you're worried that his career and earning potential will be limited. Will he be able to contribute to providing for the family? Or maybe you're worried about his mental health. Will he be depressed or demoralized by failing in his presentation?

Underneath our sometimes critical behavior is usually some vulnerability or pain that we fear. When our response is rooted in trying to avoid that pain, it usually doesn't go well.

> Fear of vulnerability or pain is often underneath critical behavior, but when we try to avoid that pain, things don't usually go well.

However, when we root our response in love rather than fear, we can hold our concern in the context of how much we love the other person. We can see his strengths. For instance, you may see how prepared your partner is for his presentation or how much he knows about the topic, and then you can rest in the knowledge that his preparation and expertise will carry the day for him. He doesn't need to be perfect to succeed. Or, if he asks you how his outfit looks, you can let him know that you really love the way the blue pants look on him and that with all his preparation and expertise, he'll be awesome. There is actually no need to focus on what he lacks. Rather, when you hold and highlight his strengths, he is more likely to succeed.

Just as kind coaches get more out of their athletes by noticing where they could do better, holding that in the context of their particular strengths, and encouraging them, so too do we and our partners do better when we feel loved and encouraged. We might think of the message of someone needing improvement as the strong back. It takes courage to speak up and let our partners know we need something different. But when we do it without the soft front, our partners can feel like they've been clubbed with a stick. Adding in the vulnerability of the soft front makes all the difference. To do so, we must see the vulnerability of our partners and hold them in the context of love and caring. And we must also learn to speak to them out of our own vulnerability. We must own our pain and our needs rather than focusing on their shortcomings.

TRY THIS
Finding Vulnerability Underneath Criticism

Audio Track 3

Recall again the situation in which you tried to fix someone dear to you and reflect on the following:

- Why do I want to fix them?
- Do they need to be fixed?
- What is happening in me?
- Is there something that is making me feel more vulnerable than I like?
- Is there something I'm afraid of?

It's normal to have fears and to feel vulnerable, but it isn't always comfortable.

Can you stay with your discomfort a bit longer?

And then, without needing to throw yourself away and become someone different, can you meet the person you are now, fears and all, and begin to explore what would help you right now by offering yourself kindness? Ask:

- Is there something that I can do to reassure myself?

What would you say to a friend who had the same fear or was feeling vulnerable? How would you reassure your friend?

Can you say the same things to yourself right now? Stay with it for as long as you need.

When your own physiology has eased a bit, turn your attention toward your partner:

- What would happen if I spoke to my partner out of love rather than fear?
- What would I say?
- How would that be for me?
- How would that be for my partner?
- What impact might it have on my relationship?

In this way we begin to see how we can work with pain and vulnerability—our own and our partner's. This sets the stage for being able to get things done from a place of responsiveness rather than reactivity. We'll explore more about this other way of working with it in the next chapter. For now, it's enough to know that changes and improvements do need to happen. Fixing, controlling, and criticizing are common strategies we use when we are resisting opening to the pain of the threat/defense system. We often attempt to use the drive system to avoid pain.

Try noticing when you start fixing, controlling, or criticizing. Realizing that we are moving into the drive system as a way to *avoid pain* rather than as a response to pain gives us the opportunity to move toward our pain and give ourselves the support we need so that we have the capacity to stay connected.

Luckily, we have a system that is designed to help us hold ourselves and each other when we are in pain. In the next chapter we turn our attention to the care system and how learning to tend to ourselves and our partners in this system changes everything.

4

"Do You Care?"

Finding Safe Connection

The only thing we never get enough of is love; and the only thing we never give enough of is love.

—HENRY MILLER

"I know what you want. You need me to shut up and drive," he said. And in that moment I knew I was safe with him. It was very early in the morning, and we were on our way to the hospital where I was to have surgery. There was a period in my life when I had a variety of difficult health challenges. During this time, I had several surgeries and other procedures. Unfortunately, they didn't always go well, and I was injured by the people who were tasked with helping me. Going under anesthesia is a very vulnerable situation. It disables both the threat/defense system with its ability to fight or flee and the drive system with its ability to find solutions to the problem. When we are vulnerable like this, we are completely dependent on the care we receive from others. We need to know other people are tuned in to us and will notice our distress, show up, and tend to our safety.

Having been injured in the past meant I was dealing with a bit of past trauma in addition to the normal anxiety of preparing for surgery. My sympathetic nervous system was very activated in response to the perceived threat. The sympathetic nervous system is like the gas in a car. It gives us the energy to fight or flee. Neither of those strategies would be helpful to me here. I knew I needed the surgery. Luckily, there is another system—our parasympathetic nervous system—which is like the brakes in a car. It's what slows down the activation of the sympathetic nervous system and helps us feel calmer, safer, and more at ease. I knew what to do to activate the parasympathetic nervous system, and I was deeply engaged in practices to comfort and calm myself. It wasn't visible from the outside. I just seemed quiet.

And that was a difficult situation for my husband. He was scared too—after all, his wife was about to have surgery. In the past, he'd avoided his anxiety by taking work calls while we were in pre-op. As you can imagine, that didn't go over so well. After that he also tried engaging me in small talk, which I found a burden, as if I needed to take care of him and his anxiety. And, of course, he tried talking with me about the plan for making me better, but that also felt like a distraction. It had us skipping over the scary situation I was currently in. As I had explained to him in the past, what I really needed was just to be held. Not physically, as that would be hard to do while driving, but emotionally. I didn't need him to say anything. I just needed to know that he knew how I felt and that he was there for me, tuned in and ready to help with whatever I needed. I needed to know that he would *follow my lead,* rather than *lead me* wherever he imagined might be helpful. I needed his loving, connected presence.

So when he said that I just needed him to "shut up and drive," I felt seen, heard, connected, safe, and loved. For the record, I'd never asked him to "shut up." That seemed a bit harsh to me. But I appreciated that it was his way of underlining that he understood that he needed to stop filling the space with words and instead just be present with me. Whatever was to come, I knew I had an ally who would not be under anesthesia. And that made a huge difference to me.

The Care System

What was happening between us isn't unusual. It is a manifestation of how the care system works so beautifully. It took me from my own activated threat/defense system and comforted and soothed me so that I could safely engage in fixing the problem with my drive system. We often need help calming our physiology so that we can move into whatever it is we need to do. Life is a balance between doing and being. As the saying goes, we are not "human doings," we are "human beings." We need to learn to be with ourselves and each other as we are. That very ability to be, when done in a caring context, is what allows us to then do what we need to do from a place of calm and safety. I felt safer when my husband was able to be with me while I was in distress. I knew I wasn't facing it alone, and my physiology relaxed a bit.

Paul Gilbert, the developer of compassion-focused therapy, talks about this as the third emotion regulation system, the care system. As mammals, our young are born very vulnerable, and it takes a long time for them to mature. Without someone taking care of them, our infants would die and our species wouldn't survive. Luckily, we are physiologically wired to care for each other. The baby smiles and coos, and we are charmed and attentive. The baby cries, and we are distressed. We are motivated to find and alleviate the source of the infant's distress. Often this takes the form of holding and rocking the baby as we sing or talk sweetly. According to Gilbert, when we are in the care system (which he also calls the *soothing and affiliation system*), we experience feelings of peaceful well-being, contentment, "safeness," and connection that help to open our attention and soften anxiety. It allows us to reason and reflect in more positive and gentler ways and directs behavior toward slower, calmer actions.

Especially when we are vulnerable, we need to know we are safely connected. We need to know that someone will be there to care for us, whether that means nurturing us with food and love, protecting us by providing shelter and standing up for us, or comforting and soothing us when we are in distress. And how does that soothing actually happen? It happens through affiliation. When we feel safely and securely connected to someone else, we can relax a bit. We can trust that someone else will help us when we need help.

TRY THIS
Feeling Safely Connected

Think about a time you felt safely connected to someone. Maybe it was a grandparent, a pet, a therapist, or a dear friend. It could even be your partner.

Allow yourself to feel their presence now. As you pause to hang out with them, just enjoy their good company. Stay here as long as you like.

Notice what is happening to you physically, emotionally, and mentally when you bathe in their kind presence.

It's likely that when you remember feeling safely connected, your threat/defense system quiets down and you begin to feel safe, calm, and connected. You experience a sense of safeness.

The care system is characterized by feeling safe, connected, and content. This contentment is very different than the pleasure we seek through our drive system. Where the drive system is activating and has us searching for hits of dopamine, the care system doesn't have the same activation. Here we feel calm and content. We don't need to pursue anything to be well. The hormones in the care system are oxytocin, often called the "love hormone," and endorphins. Endorphins are also helpful in reducing pain.

One study in particular stands out to me as providing evidence for the power of the care system. Researchers looked at the role of touch in reducing pain and enabling one person in a couple to accurately feel the other's emotions. They used the brain imaging tool of fMRI so they could see what was happening in the brains of the person in pain and in the person's partner simultaneously. What they found was that when the partner touched the person in pain, the partner more accurately perceived their partner's pain and that very touch was associated with pain reduction for the person experiencing the pain. And these effects were stronger with a romantic partner than they were with a stranger. That's quite a study. Touch is one of the avenues for compassion, as we will explore in Part II of this book. What the results of this study mean is that the physical connection of touch can help us be more accurate in perceiving

> Touch helps us perceive our partner's pain more accurately—and connection through touch can actually reduce our experience of pain.

our partners' pain *and* that very connection through touch can actually reduce our experience of pain.

Compassion for ourselves and compassion for our partners are both care system activities. The ideal way to learn self-compassion is, of course, through receiving compassion from others. In psychotherapy the presence of the therapist is everything. Study after study concludes that the *relationship* between the therapist and the patient is more predictive of positive treatment outcomes than the actual modality of treatment.

Compassion teachers experience the same thing. The power of teaching comes from the teacher's embodying compassion while teaching. We teach self-compassion by embodying compassion for our participants. By treating them with compassion, we are modeling how they can begin to treat themselves with the same kindness. It is a transmission of compassion through the relationship between the student and the teacher.

When we are treated with kindness and compassion by our parents, our therapists, our friends, and our partners, we implicitly understand and tend toward compassion for ourselves. Know that when you treat your partner with the kindness and compassion of the care system, you are literally laying down the foundation for your partner to develop self-compassion.

Far different from the "fixing" that is often the focus in the drive system, here the culture of care is the impetus for healing. We aren't necessarily trying for a particular outcome. We are just attending to the person who is struggling. In doing so, we increase the safety of the other person. We can increase his, her, or their safety through the care system's strong-back activities (providing, protecting, and motivating) or through its soft-front activities (comforting, validating, and soothing). Often, there is a combination of the two.

As Paul Gilbert notes, we know we are in the care system when we feel safe, content, and connected. This system is underutilized and underdeveloped in our culture. It helps to balance the activation of the threat/defense and drive systems. Engaging the care system can change everything when we or our partners are in distress. Our own experience improves, our partners' experience improves, and our relationships improve. When the care system in our relationships is active, we feel safe in our relationships, we feel connected, and we can be vulnerable with each other. That very vulner-

> The vulnerability made possible by the safety of being in the care system can help partners become more fully themselves and is the foundation of all successful relationships.

ability, now possible because of the increased safety in the relationship, creates the intimacy between partners, and it is also what helps both people become more fully themselves. It is the foundation of all successful relationships.

The Role of Compassion

Compassion is a response to suffering. When we are struggling, it is the desired response. Rather than co-opting the drive system to help us get out of pain, as we explored in Chapter 3, what we need is actually to activate the care system. Compassion is a function of the care system. It's how we take care of each other and ourselves when we are struggling. To begin, let's look at compassion through the lens of the strong back and soft front, as we have been doing throughout the book.

Strong Back: Provide, Protect, and Motivate

We benefit from others using their strong back to help us. We can think of the strong back as providing, protecting, and motivating us with strength. In our early days, our caregivers go out into the world to bring back resources for us. We need food, clothing, and shelter. As children, we are not yet able to get these things for ourselves, so our caregivers provide them for us. In other words, they use their strength to provide for us. In our adult relationships, we use our strengths together to provide for each other, whether that is in a primary relationship context or a work context, for example. In my case, my husband was driving the car to get me to the hospital. In addition to caring for me emotionally, he was physically providing transport for me so I didn't have to find my own way there. That was strong-back compassion. He was providing for me. It is easy for this aspect to be taken for granted, but it actually freed me up to tend to myself emotionally.

Protection is another aspect of the strength of the care system. As I write this, I have the image of how my children used to hide behind my legs when they were little and felt frightened. There is a sense that our caregivers will protect us from harm. When we are little, we can't do that for ourselves. And beyond protecting us from physical harm, our loved ones can help protect us from emotional harm as well. When someone is being bullied, it helps a great deal when a person witnessing the bullying steps in and says that bullying isn't right and needs to stop. This is as true when we are little and need the adults to stop a sibling from picking on us as it is today, when thousands are marching and demanding an end to systemic oppression and the killing of people of color. We need to stand in solidarity with each other to stop harm. We need to protect each other. The more people stand up for protection, the safer we all become. It really helps to have an ally who will protect us, as well as they can. Knowing my husband would be looking out for me while I couldn't protect myself was a great comfort.

The third aspect of the strong back of compassion is motivation. We can use our connections to motivate and encourage others to go out into the world and achieve their goals. Think about that word, *encourage. En* means to make or put in. So when we combine *en* with *courage*, we put courage into the other person. We might think of it as lending our courage to another, whether that is through holding out our hands to the baby who is ready to take her first steps or leaving our young adult at college with reassurance that this new college student will be fine and this is the beginning of an exciting time, or encouraging our partners as they prepare to give a big presentation at work. We can lend them our strength and give them the confidence they need to grow in their own strength and abilities. Ultimately this encouragement we provide can lead to our partners being able to become the fullest expression of themselves.

Finding the Strong Back of Compassion

Audio Track 5

Remember a time when you were scared—not a time when something traumatic was happening; instead please choose something easier to work with here. Maybe you got a bad review at work or your partner was unhappy with you. Maybe you experienced subtle discrimination because of your age, gender identity, sexual orientation, or racial identity.

Could you lean on anyone for help?

- If so, what did the person do that was helpful?
- Can you feel the strength of compassion in the way that person stood up for you (protected), gave you what you needed to get through it (provided), or encouraged you to make a change (motivated)?

If no one was there for you to lean on, and even if there was, can you now feel into your own strong back?

How might you take steps to protect yourself, provide for yourself, or motivate yourself?

What would a loved one say to you or what would you say to a loved one?

Can you try saying those things to yourself?

Perhaps try freely and spontaneously writing a letter of support to yourself.

When you are done, take some time to read through it. Can you feel yourself being strengthened by your own strong back?

Notice the two avenues to activating the care system through your strong back: compassion from others and compassion from yourself. Both are relational. Which do you prefer? Is there room for both?

Soft Front: Comfort, Validate, Soothe

On the other side of things is the soft front of vulnerability. Our kind and caring presence can make it safe for our loved ones to be vulnerable through comfort, validation, and soothing. Again, I think of when my children were little. When they were injured, they'd crawl into my lap for comfort and reassurance. I'd usually say something like "It's okay. I'm right here." I was tapping into the power of the affiliative system to provide safety. Not that I knew that at the time. At the time it was just instinctive. We are wired this way.

Even in adulthood—when we are ill, for example—it makes a big difference if someone tends to us by fluffing our pillow, bringing a warm blanket, or offering a cup of tea. These things tend to make us feel safe and comforted, and we can relax a bit. There are also times when we need to be validated. Maybe we are facing a difficult conversation. It helps when someone is there to reassure us by validating that we are seeing clearly, we should speak up, and we'll be okay. When we find ourselves brokenhearted, having someone dear to us hold us while we cry, listen to our stories of brokenheartedness, or offer us poetry, tissues, stories, and most of all their kind presence is very soothing. We can think of comfort as physical compassion, validation as mental compassion, and soothing as emotional compassion.

The Vulnerability of the Soft Front Is Foundational for Intimacy

As adults we still need comfort, validation, and soothing. And we can't get these without being vulnerable. We need to admit to ourselves and to our partners that we are having a difficult time. We often get stuck here. We need to be loved through our difficulty, but we can't admit we need that. We are afraid to be vulnerable. When we are afraid to be vulnerable, we may look for these things in substances instead of people. We may feel like we need to have a drink or some junk food, or to binge-watch Netflix, for example. Too many of us have lost our way with how we can best be soothed, comforted, and reassured. Substances are a poor substitute for affiliation.

Brené Brown, a researcher who studies shame resilience, talks about how we need to allow ourselves to be truly, deeply seen to be loved. This is a vulnerable situation for us. What if you see me and you don't like me? We are vulnerable *because* of our need to belong. To allow ourselves to be comforted via affiliation involves being vulnerable. We need to open to the pain that we are in. Admitting to ourselves or our loved ones that we are actually in pain right now doesn't make us weak. It makes us courageous. It can be scary to face the truth of our vulnerability, especially in our relationships.

> Admitting to our pain is not a sign of weakness but of courage.

If we think being vulnerable will make us unattractive to our partners, then we may resist being vulnerable with them. We may also resist sharing our vulnerability if we don't trust them to be there for us when we need them. This is why one of relationship expert John Gottman's core skills is turning toward our partners when they make a bid for our attention.

Brené Brown also talks about the vulnerability paradox: I feel safer when you are vulnerable with me, but not when I'm vulnerable with you. For the care system to work well, both of us need to be vulnerable with each other. Vulnerability is at the core of intimacy. One thing that can help us open to being vulnerable with our partners, so that they have a chance of comforting, soothing, and validating us, is the practice of self-compassion. (We'll explore that more fully in Part II of this book.) The other thing that can help us open to vulnerability is the way our partners receive us when we share our difficulty with them.

TRY THIS

Finding the Soft Front of Compassion

Audio Track 6

Think about a time when you were feeling vulnerable. Maybe you failed, felt inadequate, or were otherwise suffering in some way. Not the most difficult situation you've ever been in, nothing traumatic. Something easier, like maybe you had the flu, failed a test, or missed a goal so your team lost the game.

Can you feel the pain of it? Could you let yourself feel it at the time?

Could you let anyone know you were having a difficult time?

- If not, what got in the way?

Was anyone there to comfort, reassure, or soothe you in some way?

- If so, what did you find helpful? Touch, a kind gaze, or gentle words?

If no one was there for you to lean on, and even if someone was, can you now feel into your own soft front?

- Can you allow yourself to know your vulnerability?

How might you take steps to comfort, reassure, or soothe yourself?

- What would a loved one say to you, or what would you say to a loved one?
- Can you try saying those things to yourself?

Or perhaps try freely and spontaneously writing a letter of support to yourself.

When you are done, take some time to read through it. Can you feel yourself safely held and cared for in the vulnerability of your soft front?

Notice the two avenues to activating the care system through your soft front: compassion from others and compassion from yourself. Both are relational. Which do you prefer? Is there room for both?

We have now looked at the care system through a few lenses. We've explored how it developed because we are born vulnerable and how affiliation is the best route to our survival. We've looked at it through the strong back and the soft front. And we've noticed that we can take an interpersonal approach (receiving care from others) and an intrapersonal approach (receiving care from ourselves). We'll look more closely at those two approaches later in the book. Now let's look at an example of how the care system functions well in helping couples support each other in difficult times.

Sam and Susie: From Fixing to Care

I had been seeing Sam and Susie in couples therapy for some time. There were a variety of issues, and they were pretty cut off from each other emotionally. Yet they had a family together, and they really wanted to make the relationship work—if only *the other* would be vulnerable first. One day I got a text from Susie. She wanted to let me know that her biopsy was positive. She had cancer. I called her back right away, and as I held the diagnosis with her, she mentioned I was the first person she had called. A few days later Susie and Sam were in my office for a session. Things were really difficult for them. Sam was upset that he wasn't the first person Susie had called.

Susie was also upset. She explained that when Sam found out he immediately went into "fix-it mode." He called in all of his connections to find the best treatment center for her. He got a copy of the pathology report and consulted with family and friends who were doctors about the type of cancer she had, the available treatments, and the prognosis. He let her know that her prognosis looked good. He was like a tornado of "helpfulness." Only Susie wasn't finding it helpful at all. Quite the opposite, she felt simultaneously bombarded and discarded. She felt like a broken toy that needed to be fixed. She wondered if he would discard her if it turned out she wasn't easy to fix. She needed some space to breathe and feel her feelings before deciding on her course of action. She was scared. What Susie needed first was for Sam to hold the scary feelings with her. That way she wouldn't be alone with them.

I pointed out to Sam that he'd gone into fixing mode. I wondered what was underneath that fixing mode and what vulnerable feelings had been activated. To his credit, he was able to redirect toward his vulnerable feelings. He explained how scared he was of losing Susie, how she was the center of his life and how, having recently lost a parent, he didn't think he could bear another loss. As Sam landed more fully in his own fear, Susie finally felt permission to talk about her own fear. Her fear of dying, her fear of treatment, her fear of being too much for Sam and how she feared he might discard her—it all came tumbling out. This time, instead of fixing Susie, Sam was able to be present with her. He comforted her as he looked into her eyes and reassured her that he wasn't leaving and he'd be there for her. I could see the effects on both of them. Their bodies softened and they leaned closer together as he held her hand. They shared some tears. It was still a difficult path ahead, but they now had each other. Sam softened when Susie explained that she had waited to tell him because she was afraid he'd go into fixing mode. Sam now knew what Susie really needed. She needed him, his presence, his strength, and his reassurance. She needed his vulnerability *and* his strength. She needed his caring.

The Right System at the Right Time

As Sam and Susie illustrate, each of the three systems (threat/defense, drive, and care) can be helpful at times; however, the order in which we engage the systems makes a big difference in our relationships.

Safety First: The Role of the Threat/Defense System

Remember that whenever we feel threatened, the threat/defense system is dominant. This is why many theorists note that safety is a precondition for compassion to arise. "If your heart is a volcano," wrote Khalil Gibran, "how shall you expect flowers to bloom?" When we are caught in the threat/defense system, our heart often feels like a volcano. This is the system that was activated for both Susie and Sam when Susie received a life-threatening diagnosis. The system is actually designed for acute threats like this. It is an activating system, triggered so that Susie will do something about the threat to her life. However, in relationships we can find ourselves chronically in the threat/defense system. If you find yourself frequently angry, disgusted, or anxious in your relationship, it is likely that you and your relationship are lacking in safety and caught in the threat/defense mode. In this system we are reactive rather than responsive. This happens because the amygdala is activated and the frontal cortex—which helps us reason and respond—is deactivated. In other words, our access to wisdom is blocked.

Being stuck in this mode is really painful. It certainly doesn't lead to the blossoming of the relationship. Instead we find ourselves more and more discouraged and despondent. Buddha is quoted as saying, "Hatred does not cease by hatred, but only by love; this is the eternal rule." Sometimes being stuck in the threat/defense system is characterized by chronic anger and fighting. Other times it is more distant, fueled by withdrawing or even by placating. Whichever is the case, we certainly don't feel safe being vulnerable with our partners when we are stuck in this system.

Physiologically the threat/defense system dominates whenever we feel unsafe. This is as it should be. When our very survival is at risk, the threat/defense system activities of fight, flight, and freeze are appropriately protective. For example, those who have found themselves on the battlefield are taught to fight. Or if fighting is not possible, to withdraw (flee). And if that isn't possible, then to surrender (freeze). These actions are literally lifesaving. Similarly, if you find yourself in a domestic violence situation, this threat/defense system may be lifesaving. Depending on your circumstances in any given moment, it may be wise to fight, flee, or freeze. (If you are in this situation, please reach out for help. Your life matters. There are resources at the end of this book to point you in the right direction.) In the order of things, safety always comes first.

As you can see, the threat/defense system is key to our survival. It is the dominant system because we are wired to put safety first. In situations that threaten your life, it would be foolish to sit with a hand on your heart, note that this is a stressful situation, and say kind words to yourself. In our modern world, however, it's more common to experience threats to how we feel than to our survival, and the threat/defense system doesn't serve us well relationally.

Trying to Get Rid of Pain by Activating the Drive System

None of us like to be in pain, emotional or otherwise. We want to be happy, and we think the path to happiness is through ridding ourselves of pain. We call up one of the drive system strategies—fixing, controlling, or criticizing—to solve our problems. But as we explored in Chapter 3, this approach doesn't work out well for us in our relationships. When we are in pain, we don't want our partners to fix, control, or criticize us. The use of fixing, controlling, or criticizing is meant to restore safety, but it actually makes the relationship more and more unsafe for both people.

This may be due in part to the fact that we are trying to activate the drive system for purposes it wasn't designed to serve. Paul Gilbert would say in fact that the *real* drive system isn't rooted in avoidance of pain. It is designed strictly to get things done. Although we may not realize it at the time, underneath our attempts to fix, control, or criticize, we ourselves are in pain and actually still in our threat/defense system. We tap the drive system in the hope of solving the "problem" of being in pain, but all that really accomplishes is to burden us with tasks to make the pain go away. This is really a form of resistance to our pain, and because what we resist tends to grow stronger, this use of the drive system actually makes things worse. We are thus stuck in an activation of both the drive and threat/defense systems. In our attempt to become *safer*, we, our partners, and our relationships actually become *less* safe emotionally. So where *do* we find happiness?

Safeness through Connection: The Care System

Rather than trying to get rid of our pain, when we open to it and meet ourselves and each other with kindness and compassion we feel safer. The care system is characterized by feelings of safeness, connection, and contentment. The magic is actually in the affiliation of the care system. As noted in Chapter 1, our capacity to care for each other is what actually helps us survive as a society. I recently watched a TEDx talk in which someone asked an anthropologist what the first sign of a civilization is. She explained that it's human remains with thigh bones that have broken and healed. We can't survive after an injury like that without others to care for us while we heal. Civilization is defined in part by social organization—people caring for one another. The fundamental importance of mutual care and connection can also be seen in attachment theory, which describes how critical a safe connection to caregivers is to us early in life, not just to feed and keep us warm but to enable us to form healthy relationships throughout life. Many couples therapies, such as emotion-focused therapy, follow up on this understanding in adult life by helping couples heal their relationships by developing a secure attachment. When connection with others increases our sense of safety, we know we are in the care system. And that increased safeness of the care system actually allows us to face the truth of the painful situation we are in and gives us the resources to get through difficult times. Happiness, it turns out, is not the absence of pain but the presence of safe others who help us face the inevitable pains in life.

> Happiness is not the absence of pain but the presence of safe others who help us face the pain.

If, rather than striving to get rid of our pain by recruiting the drive system, we acknowledge the pain and accept it as the present reality and then resource ourselves through self-compassion or compassion from others, our physiology shifts. The frontal cortex, which we might call the "thinking brain" because it helps us reason and see the bigger picture of things, including consequences, can come back online. Remember that when we are in the threat/defense system this part of our brain has gone offline. When we feel safer and our physiology recovers, we again have access to the "thinking brain." Additionally, since we haven't denied or avoided the problem, we are still aware of the problem. And we now have the safety that gives us the capacity to hold the problem along with our "thinking brain" and the courage to find resources and solve problems more effectively. *Now* we are ready to utilize the drive system in the way it's meant to be used. We can pull together and work as a team to accomplish our goals. Good connection *restores* safety and makes healing possible.

TRY THIS

Moving from Drive to Care

Think about an instance when a loved one was having a difficult time and needed the protection of the threat/defense system. Not a time when the person's life was in danger. Rather, a time when your loved one was struggling with a difficult situation and the difficult feelings associated with that situation.

How did you approach the situation?

- Did you try to solve the problem so that you or your loved one could get out of pain?
- Did you try to fix the problem—telling your loved one what to do to solve it?
- Did you criticize—pointing out where your loved one was going wrong in hopes that the person would make a change that solved the problem?
- Did you control the situation by taking charge and ensuring that things were done in a way that would prevent them from getting worse and hopefully make them better?
- Can you see how you may have recruited the drive system in the hopes of *avoiding or getting rid of pain*?
- Did it make the situation better or worse?

Or maybe you simply had the wisdom to meet your loved one where they were with kindness and understanding.

In what ways did that kindness and understanding find expression?

- A kind gaze?
- Some kind touch?
- Or maybe there were some reassuring and comforting words you offered?

Did this make the situation better or worse?

Now consider a time when *you* were having a difficult time and needed the protection of the threat/defense system. Not a time when you were physically in danger. Rather, a time when you were feeling scared, lonely, or frustrated, for example. Perhaps you felt overwhelmed and all alone. Maybe you were feeling disconnected from someone you care about. Can you feel the pain of the situation?

In your heart of hearts, how would you like your partner to

respond? Rather than having your partner take over and solve the problem for you, what would have helped you to feel supported, validated, comforted, and soothed?

Can you remember a time when someone did show up for you in this way?

What happened next?

Did you feel supported enough to find a solution or otherwise begin to address your problem?

Reflecting on this exercise, notice what you would like to cultivate more of.

As we discovered above, each of the three systems is important. We do need all of them, and together they work much better if we move from the threat/defense system into the care system and hang out there for a while. After our physiology has a chance to settle and we are feeling safety, connection, and contentment, we have a much better chance of being able to use the real drive system to accomplish our goals. When we just move between the threat/defense and drive systems we may end up feeling hopelessly stuck. Typically, we already have well-developed threat/defense and drive systems; it's the care system that is underdeveloped and underutilized. If we want the true well-being of contentment, connection, and safeness, we'll need to develop and utilize the care system. There is safety when we are in the presence of kind others.

The Safety of the Care System Sets You Up to Flourish

Safety is not only a precondition for compassion; it is a precondition for flourishing. If your life is being threatened, there is not time for, and no point in, making art, for example. If interacting with your partner leaves you feeling discouraged, defeated, hopeless, worthless, and unlovable, how on earth would you have the capacity to flourish in the world—never mind flourishing in the relationship? As the poet

Mary Oliver writes, "What is it you plan to do with your one wild and precious life?" Will you spend it trying to survive your relationship, or are you in a relationship that will give you the support and confidence to pursue your dreams? Not feeling supported yet? The rest of this book looks at how we can build skills to create a more loving relationship. Feeling supported already? The rest of this book looks at how to develop the skills to build on the support you already have— deepening and strengthening your relationship and ultimately setting the stage for flourishing.

To put the function of the systems more plainly, we go from seeking safety in the threat/defense system to finding safety through affiliation, to human flourishing, as the diagram below shows.

For far too many of us, safe connection is the missing link in this system. Without it we never reach flourishing. That's why the rest of this book is on how we can cultivate the care system for ourselves, our partners, and our relationships. If we want to foster the conditions for flourishing, we must attend to loving connection.

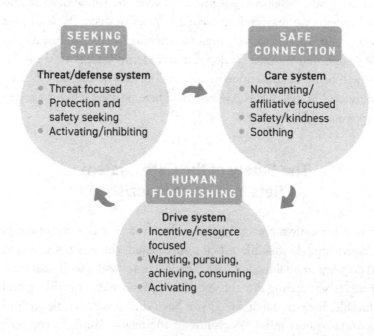

5

"Who Will Love Me?"

Ensuring That Compassion Is Always Available to You

> Having compassion starts and ends with having compassion for all those unwanted parts of ourselves. The healing comes from letting there be room for all of this to happen: room for grief, for relief, for misery, for joy.
>
> —PEMA CHÖDRÖN

To be truly, fully in the care system our relationships need to include compassion for both ourselves and our partners. Of course in healthy relationships we also receive compassion from our partners. As you may have discovered in the preceding chapters, most of us have blocks to being as fully compassionate as we would like. The really good news is that compassion is a skill that can be cultivated! That's just where we are headed now.

That poses a question, though. Do we practice compassion for ourselves or our partners first? Most of us already know how to be compassionate to others, but many of us have trouble taking care of our own needs. As young girls many of us women were sold the "Cinderella complex." Our fairy tales led us to believe that Prince Charming would come along and complete us. Men, who learn by age five not to be like their mothers—to reject vulnerability and other soft feelings and needs—wish to have a wife who will take care of their vulnerable selves and meet their needs for intimacy. Luckily, our culture is

changing, and these notions are becoming outdated as such qualities are no longer limited to a particular gender—even gender itself is
becoming more fluid, or at least our awareness of it is. Still, there is a
notion that we will find the one to "complete us," and together we will
find wholeness. This is a tricky situation that leaves us feeling dependent on a partner to meet our needs. Dependency breeds resentment
in both partners—the one whose needs go unmet and the one who
feels solely responsible for meeting the partner's needs. This isn't ideal
for anyone.

As I often say to my patients, it is better to be in a relationship
because we *want* to be in the relationship than because we *need* to
be in the relationship. When we *need* to be in a relationship, we are
willing to tolerate things we shouldn't be tolerating. We hitch our own
survival to the survival of the relationship.

However, when we learn to meet our own needs, when we can
comfort and soothe ourselves, we are no longer dependent on a partner. We always have access to what we need, even when a partner isn't
available to us. One way to do this is to learn self-compassion.

One of the reasons our partners aren't available to us, as we
explored in earlier chapters, is that they may be caught in their threat/
defense system. The same is true for us. When we ourselves are caught
in our threat/defense system, it isn't possible to be there for our partners. This is another reason we need to have a strong self-compassion
practice. When we can meet ourselves with compassion, we can move
from threat/defense to our care system, and when we do we become
available to engage in compassion for our partners. That's why we are
starting with self-compassion. And the good news is that it doesn't
require our partners to change, something we have little power over.
We can improve our situation ourselves!

When I'm teaching compassion, I find for some people there is
resistance or even panic when I suggest they practice self-compassion.
People think I am asking them to give up on getting love from others
or that they are somehow shutting the door on receiving love from
others. To be clear, I am not suggesting anything of the kind. The
truth is that others, for whatever reason, aren't always available to
meet our needs. If we pin our hopes solely on receiving love from

others, or we are *depending* on receiving love from others, we are in a terrible position when, for whatever reason, they fail us. Other people will inevitably let us down, whether they want to or not. After all, we are all human. We get sick, we go to sleep, and we go on vacation, for example. We just cannot always be there, even for our beloveds, as much as we may want to be there for them.

Should we go without because our partners are unwilling or unable to care for us? Of course not! Rather than going without, the answer lies in going within. Once we reach adulthood, we ourselves have the capacity to provide comfort and soothing whenever we need it. Within each of us is the capacity to tend to our own needs. And the good news is that we are each the one person we have access to 24/7. I'm talking here about the importance of developing a self-compassion practice.

It sounds so easy, doesn't it? Once the practice is established, it truly is easy. But the road there can be bumpy. It's common to feel a profound sadness when we see the ways in which we've been trying to cope with not having our needs met. And, of course, there's an overwhelming sadness as we see the bigger picture of not having had enough of our needs met. This sadness isn't a problem. If we let it, it can be the first step in truly seeing and acknowledging our own needs. Please know that you aren't alone in this and it isn't your fault. This is a normal outcome of imperfect beings doing their best to cope with imperfect circumstances. We're all just doing our best to find safety and loving connection.

Self-Compassion Practice: Always Having What You Need

With self-compassion we can begin the process of healing from the pain of unmet needs. We can develop the very same skills we would have had if we'd had a childhood with caregivers who were more attuned to our needs or an adult relationship with a partner who was more attuned to our needs. This starts with learning how to tend to our own needs in a healthy way. Only when we are healthy enough as individuals can we come together and form a relationship that is healthy. To tolerate taking the risk of being vulnerable in our relationships, as intimacy requires, we need to know that we will be okay, even if the other person can't be there for us and we come away feeling disappointed. Self-compassion gives us the confidence to show up in such a way. Even if everyone else lets us down, we aren't out of luck.

> Self-compassion gives us the confidence to be vulnerable, because we know we'll be okay even if the other person can't be there for us.

So what is self-compassion anyway? Simply put, it is treating ourselves with the same care and understanding we would offer to someone else we care about. In fact, let's pause here and take a moment to really see how this typically plays out in our lives.

TRY THIS

Discovering How We Treat Ourselves and Others

Audio Track 7

Take a moment to remember a time or various times when a dear friend (not your partner) was having a really hard time. Maybe your friend got some difficult feedback at work, or just received a difficult health diagnosis, or perhaps your friend was having a relational problem with a partner, child, or sibling.

How do you typically respond?

- What do you say?
- What tone do you use? Is it soft and warm? Or is it cold and harsh?
- What words do you use?
- Is there any physical gesture of kindness?

Take a moment and note how you typically treat your good

friends when they are having a hard time. You may even want to write down what you found.

Now take a moment to remember a time or various times when you were having a really hard time. Maybe your boss gave you some difficult feedback, you just received a difficult health diagnosis, or you felt concerned about or let down by a child, partner, or sibling.

How do you typically respond to yourself in such situations?

- What do you say to yourself?

- Is your tone warm or harsh?

- What words do you use?

- Is there any physical gesture of kindness?

Take a moment and note how you typically respond to yourself when you are having a hard time. If you like, you can write this down too.

Now take a moment to remember a time or various times when your partner was having a difficult time. Maybe your partner got some painful feedback at work, a difficult health diagnosis, or was in the midst of a relational problem with a child, sibling, or even with you.

How do you typically respond to your partner when your partner is having a difficult time?

- What do you say?

- Is your tone kind or critical?

- What words do you typically use?

- Is there any physical gesture of kindness?

Take a moment to note how you typically respond to your partner during their hard time. It is often helpful to write this down as well.

Now notice the relationship between your responses to the three different people. Where is it easiest to feel compassion? What is most challenging for you? Are they about the same?

Researcher Kristin Neff and colleagues looked at the difference in the first two scenarios. They found that the vast majority of people (78 percent) are more compassionate toward others than themselves. Sixteen percent are more equal in their compassion toward themselves and others, and only 6 percent are more compassionate toward themselves than others. Although I am not aware of research looking at compassion directed toward a partner versus ourselves, when I teach this exercise in the Compassion for Couples program, people often find that they treat their partners even worse than they treat themselves. This usually comes as a surprise.

The good news is that Neff and colleagues also conducted research that showed when people learn self-compassion they also increase positive relational behaviors and decrease negative relational behaviors. So you might say people who learn self-compassion also become kinder in their relationships. Far from turning us into narcissists, self-compassion actually helps us become better at relationships.

Self-Compassion: Mindfulness, Common Humanity, and Self-Kindness

According to Dr. Kristin Neff, the leading researcher on self-compassion, self-compassion is made up of three components: mindfulness, common humanity, and self-kindness. All three of these components have to be present at once for self-compassion to exist. In the chapters that follow we take a closer look at each of these components, especially how we can apply them in the service of developing self-compassion. For now, let's briefly explore the components the way we explore them in the mindful self-compassion (MSC) program developed by Christopher Germer and Kristin Neff.

Mindfulness

The first component in Neff's model of self-compassion is mindfulness. Many of us get caught up in the story of what is happening to us, ruminating on a problem we may have rather than seeing it in a more balanced and objective way. On the other hand, we may fail to notice that there is a problem. I like to think of mindfulness as a sort of balanced awareness that sees the truth of what is happening without making it bigger or smaller than it truly is. Mindfulness also helps us hold our awareness of the problem alongside awareness of the bigger picture of what is also true in this moment. For example, I had a problem with my knee that made it difficult to climb stairs. I could have just powered through this and put it out of my mind when I wasn't climbing stairs, but that would have kept me from seeing there was a problem and seeking appropriate treatment. Meanwhile, the problem was likely to grow worse.

> Mindfulness is balanced awareness that sees the truth without making what's happening larger or smaller than it is.

On the other hand, I could have ruminated on the pain in my knee, noting how bad it was going to be. For example, my office was on the second floor. What would happen if I could no longer make it up the stairs to my office? Was I going to have to close my practice? And what would happen to me without income? The rumination could create suffering much greater than the actual pain in my knee.

The mindful approach had me acknowledging the pain in my knee and also that I had options to treat the pain. And ultimately, if needed, I could move to a first-floor office. The mindful approach led to much less suffering than if I had tried to deny the problem or if I had overfocused on it. Let's take a moment so you can identify and work with your own tendency. I'll slowly unpack a variation of the Self-Compassion Break practice from MSC, interspersed with a deeper understanding of each component. You'll want to be sure to do all three "Try This" practices to get a sense of how to skillfully work with painful situations. (They are combined in the audio files.)

Putting Self-Compassion into Practice, Part I—Mindfulness

Audio Track 8

Bring to mind something you are in the midst of that is causing distress. Not the most stressful situation in your life; a 3–4 on the scale of distress where 10 is unbearable. Allow yourself to open fully to the situation.

As you consider the difficulty, notice where your mind goes.

- Do you tend to push the problem away or tamp it down?
- Or do you tend to make it bigger, perhaps anticipating the other problems it may cause?
- Can you come back to just the reality of what is happening in this moment?

What is happening with your emotions?

- Can you feel the feeling—sadness, fear, or whatever might be there?
- Are you pushing away the feeling?
- Or are you feeding it and making it more intense?
- See if you can find your way back to opening to the feeling, just as it is.
- Perhaps you can name the feeling.

Finally, see what is happening in your body. Often we feel a problem somewhere in the body.

- Take a moment and scan your body for where you feel it most easily. You might notice, for example, an achiness in the chest or a hollowness in the belly. Perhaps it is tightness in the throat or a hot red face.
- Take a moment to acknowledge what the body is holding.

- If you can, invite some softness into the area that is holding the tension.
- You may even offer the kindness of a hand over the part of the body that is holding the tension.

Can you allow it to be just like this for now?

Opening to our situation just like it is, without pushing it away or allowing ourselves to be carried away, can actually be a relief. When we allow things to be just as they are, we aren't saying that we agree with it or that it is okay with us. We are simply acknowledging things as they are. The body can soften, the emotions can settle, the mind can rest in the knowledge that it's like *this* right now. And we hold this along with the sense of impermanence, which reminds us not to get attached to how things are right now, as things often change.

Common Humanity

The second component in Neff's model of self-compassion is common humanity, which reminds us that these kinds of things happen to all humans. We get sick, feel rejected, fail, and so on. We are not alone in this. It is part of the shared human condition. That said, it is important to recognize that, while all beings suffer, we don't all suffer equally. Due to both systemic injustice and our individual circumstances, the degree to which we suffer isn't the same for everyone. Common humanity doesn't say we all suffer equally; it simply says all humans do suffer. However common or rare our circumstances are, there are others who are experiencing the same challenges. For example, Neff often talks about how she was struggling with her son's diagnosis of autism, what that meant for her and for him, and how her life wouldn't be the same as she had anticipated. One day she was at a playground with him and feeling the pain of being in a different situation than she'd anticipated and than the other moms were in when she realized that she actually had lots in common with the other moms. "This is what it feels like for all moms when we worry about our kids, struggle with things not being as we think they should be, or feel overwhelmed with the responsibilities of parenting." Suddenly, instead of being isolated, which Neff names as the opposite of common humanity, she was connected to all mothers everywhere. And that connectedness with others gave her the confidence that she could get through this. Let's take a more personal look at this aspect of self-compassion now.

TRY THIS

Putting Self-Compassion into Practice, Part II—Common Humanity

Audio Track 8

Bring to mind the same situation you worked with in the preceding practice.

Notice any thoughts of how things shouldn't be like this or how others are having a better experience while you are uniquely struggling. Perhaps you are having thoughts that others wouldn't understand?

What emotions are you experiencing? Perhaps there is a sense of overwhelm, hopelessness, despair, fear? See what it is for you.

Now see what happens when you broaden your perspective just a bit.

Can you remember people who have struggled with similar issues? For example, maybe you feel like the only one who doesn't feel loved in their primary relationship?

What would it be like to remember others you have known who once felt the same way you do? What about people you don't know? Might there be others who share your experience or something similar?

What if you realized that those rosy pictures you see on social media cover up the pain that others are in but don't speak about? Perhaps you can recognize the way you also don't speak about the truth of the situation you are in?

What if you broaden your perspective out even further to include people who have problems right this moment? Include people whether they are experiencing the same problem as yours or not.

Can you see that having loss, failures, and disappointments is part of life, even if they aren't present for everyone at this moment? You are not alone, even if it feels that way right now. Struggle is part of every life. Sometimes it is hard to feel the truth that we are not alone. It may feel too vulnerable to let yourself feel this right now, and you may feel resistance arise. That's okay, too. Perhaps just opening your mind to the possibility that you are not alone is enough for now.

If you can, imagine yourself surrounded by others who are also struggling right now.

- How do you imagine they might feel?
- Might they have the same or similar feelings as you do?
- Everyone you are visualizing right now actually shares the pain you are in.

You belong. You are understood. You are not alone. Together you can hold the pain of this situation.

Because we have a deep need to belong, a big part of our pain is in feeling like we are suffering alone. When we believe everyone else has a perfect life, we feel there is something wrong with us for struggling the way we are. When we realize that these struggles in life are unavoidable and that we will all struggle with something as our lives unfold, we release the added burden of blaming ourselves for our situation and feeling there is something wrong with us for feeling this way. Beyond making us feel less alone and less defective, when we recognize our shared common humanity, we belong. The heart can now open. We can get through this, just like others around us have gotten or are getting through this particular struggle. There is strength in numbers.

Self-Kindness

The third component of Neff's model of self-compassion is self-kindness. She views self-kindness as the opposite of self-criticism or self-judgment. When things aren't going well for us, how do we relate to ourselves? Many people think if they are kind to themselves they won't get anywhere, so they push themselves in a harsh and critical way in order to motivate themselves. However, the research shows just the opposite is true. Harsh self-judgment only shuts us down and makes us less able to achieve our goals. Others of us were met with harsh, critical, unkind words from our families or other important figures in our life, and we internalized these unkind messages and continue to say these harsh things to ourselves. Thinking back to the earlier exercise in this chapter that had you compare how you treat others with how you treat yourself, what did you notice? As I noted on page 84, the research suggests that 78 percent of people treat themselves worse than they treat others. It isn't because they don't know how to be kind. Rather, the fact that we treat others with kindness says we *can* be kind. We just need to practice directing kindness toward ourselves. Let's continue our practice and see what happens when we try meeting ourselves with kindness rather than self-judgment.

TRY THIS

Putting Self-Compassion into Practice, Part III—Kindness

Audio Track 8

Once again calling to mind the situation you worked with in the preceding practices, open to the pain of the situation, remembering you are not alone with it:

Can you offer yourself some gesture of kindness?

Perhaps placing your hand on the part of the body that is holding the distress as a way of offering warmth and support?

If you like, you can invite that part of the body to soften a bit, without requiring it to change—just softening around it, providing a soft place for the body to relax and release any tension that isn't currently serving you.

Stay here as long as you want.

Are there any kind words you need to hear?

Perhaps words that you would offer a dear friend who was struggling in the same way? "I'm here for you" or "You'll get through this" or "That's really rough, and it isn't your fault."

Try offering the same kind words to yourself now. You may need to say them over and over.

And, only if it feels right to you, you might try letting the words in to receive your own kindness.

Stay here as long as you want.

Before you finish this exercise, just take a moment to notice any effects of this exercise.

- How do you feel now?

- Has anything shifted?

- Which part of this was most powerful? Mindfulness? Common humanity? Self-kindness?

- Was there any part that didn't feel right?

Perhaps there was a part that felt like too much? That's okay, too. You can just take the parts that feel good to you right now.

What happened for you when you offered yourself kindness? This can be both a really big challenge and deeply healing. If it felt deeply healing, you're on your way to self-compassion. If it was challenging, don't despair. That's a common experience when we begin to learn self-compassion. We will be looking at each of these three components in more detail in the following chapters as we learn to cultivate compassion for ourselves, our partners, and our relationships. We'll be unpacking them in a slower, more approachable way, which can make all the difference.

Self-Compassion: From State to Trait

> A moment of self-compassion can change your entire day. A
> string of such moments can change the course of your life.
> —CHRISTOPHER K. GERMER

I love this thought from Chris Germer. It is so very true. What he is pointing to is that the state of self-compassion is wonderful, but the real power is in the trait of self-compassion. How do we move from experiencing the state of self-compassion to developing a way of being that is self-compassionate? By collecting a string of such moments. What we practice grows stronger. So if we practice self-criticism, or self-isolation or rumination, as many of us have spent our lifetime doing, that habit grows stronger. If instead we practice self-compassion, that habit becomes stronger, eventually becoming our default.

Over time, this practice helps us cultivate and deepen our capacity to be in the care system rather than being based in reactivity or getting caught in endless efforts to fix our problems. As Gilbert notes, in the care system we feel content, connected, and safe. Who wouldn't want to spend more time feeling this way?

How to Practice Self-Compassion

It's helpful to approach our practice as a big experiment. We are all different, and in different current circumstances, and given this, what you will need at any given time, or what will be helpful, is likely to vary from moment to moment and from person to person. Some practices will be really helpful for you, and others may not. The only way to find out is to give them a try. The program I like for learning self-compassion is the MSC program. It is the most established and well-validated program for learning self-compassion. Many of the practices I'll suggest come out of or are adapted from this program. I'll give you an intro to some of them here, but I hope you'll take the program if you want to take a deeper dive.

One of the simplest and most accessible practices I like is the practice we call *soothing or supportive touch*. We are wired to be comforted by kind touch. The good news is that we can activate our own physiology with an intentional kind touch. In the following exercise you will have a chance to experiment to find the place that works best for you.

Finding Support through Touch

Audio Track 9

Start by placing your hand on your heart. It may be helpful to close your eyes and feel into what happens in your body and what happens mentally and emotionally when you place your hand there.

Take a moment to notice the gentle pressure of the hand and perhaps the sensation of warmth.

What happens in your body when you place your hand there?

Now leave your hand there and place the other hand on your belly.

Take some time to notice what it feels like when you have your hands in this position.

Continue to experiment with what it feels like when you place your hands on different places on the body. You might try placing your hands the following ways:

- Both hands on the belly
- Cupping one or both cheeks with your hands
- Gently stroking your forearm with the opposite hand
- Stroking one or both thighs
- Placing the hands back on the heart and rubbing or tapping the heart area
- Making a fist and placing the fist over the heart area. The other hand can gently hold the fist or arm.
- Crossing your arms and giving a gentle squeeze—a surreptitious self-hug
- Holding your own hand

Take some time now just to see where your body gives you the support and reassurance you need. It could be one of these places or another—like over the throat. See where it is for you.

What happened when you tried this supportive touch? Did you find an area that was comforting and soothing? If so, it is helpful to know that this simple touch can support calming your physiology when you need it. Remember that we want to wire in things that are helpful, so if you found a spot that is helpful, please continue to use that spot intentionally at least daily. If you felt neutral about it, choose a spot and try it at least daily. Often after a few days it begins to have a positive effect. And if the kind touch really felt bad, it is a sign that this isn't right for you—at least it isn't right for you right now. There are good reasons why touch doesn't always have the desired effect. I'll talk more about that in a bit. For now, please know that I never want you to push yourself into a situation that feels harmful. How we learn self-compassion should be self-compassionate and done from a foundation of feeling safe and ready to open—never forcing yourself beyond what feels right.

Staying Safe While Practicing

We want to stay within our window of tolerance—a term coined by Dan Siegel, an expert in interpersonal neurobiology. The window of tolerance is the range of safety in which we feel able to continue to function, even if we feel a bit challenged. David Treleaven, an expert on how to practice mindfulness without triggering trauma, explains this nicely: *"When people are in their window they're more likely to feel stable, present, and regulated. When they're outside of this zone they are more likely to feel triggered, out of control, and dysregulated."*

Signs that we are no longer in the window of tolerance include too much arousal (hyperarousal) and too little arousal (hypoarousal). Treleaven goes on to describe these states:

> When we're hyperaroused, there's too much energy in the system: we can be plagued by intrusive thoughts, are anxious and easily overwhelmed, and can find it hard to relax or focus.
>
> When hypoaroused, we experience a lack of energy that leads to an absence of sensation, a lack of concentration, and a sense of immobility. . . . There, people report feeling passive, disinterested, unmotivated, and numb.

Just to be clear here, and without going full on into this important topic, hypo- and hyperarousal are how we are wired as humans. They serve important purposes, so finding yourself outside your window of tolerance doesn't mean you have done something wrong or that there is something inherently wrong with you. Rather, it usually means that we have survived difficulties in our lives that have left some residue—and that the current situation we are in isn't right for us in some way. So finding yourself outside your window of tolerance, while uncomfortable, is a sign that you need to modify what you are practicing in some way so that you feel safer.

The thing is that you get to choose what is right *for you*. Throughout this book, I offer practices to help you cultivate compassion for yourself and your partner. Depending on your own life experiences, some of these will be more skillful and effective for you to practice and others won't be as useful. One of the best ways to practice self-compassion is to customize your practice based on that quintessential question "What do I need right now?" If you find yourself outside your window of tolerance, you need to change what you are practicing or how you are practicing. As the saying goes, "less is more," and often more is less.

> Ask yourself what you need right now to adjust your self-compassion practice in order to stay within your window of tolerance.

The first place to start if you are beginning to feel mildly overwhelmed is to see if there is a way to lessen the intensity of what you are practicing. For example, when we get to the practice of cultivating loving-kindness, rather than wishing something like "May I accept myself just as I am," we can lower the dose by adding qualifiers. The more qualifiers, the lower the dose. So the phrase could become (just to exaggerate a bit) "May I begin to consider the possibility that I might eventually accept myself just as I am." Do you see how that lessens the intensity?

If the overwhelm is stronger than that, then changing the practice to something safer is often helpful. In the next chapter we will explore mindfulness practices that can help us ground in safety again. Practices like bringing our attention to an external object, like a tree, feeling the soles of our feet, or bringing our attention to the breath.

If you experience any difficulty along the way, it is likely because as we go through life difficult things happen that we may not have the resources to deal with at the time. So we scoop up the painful feelings and tuck them away. This is adaptive as it helps us to go on with our lives. Then when we have a chance to open the door of the heart to let self-compassion in, those painful experiences come tumbling out. In other words, now that we are opening to our experiences, we may find there is some pain lingering there. It can feel overwhelming or discouraging when we experience pain while giving ourselves compassion. This is what is referred to as backdraft in the MSC program. Often it seems as if something has gone wrong. However, it isn't a sign that something has gone wrong. It's actually a sign that we are finally getting what we need. It is also a sign that the dose is too big. Just like when starting an antidepressant you don't start at the effective dose, instead starting at the dosage your body can tolerate and gradually increasing the dose as it can tolerate more, in self-compassion practice we want to start with a dose that doesn't trigger difficulty for us. So please take your time and go slowly through these practices, as needed. You can always return to things you skipped whenever you feel ready. Over time you'll find you've developed a deep and sustainable practice that you can rely on whenever you feel distressed.

Learning how to treat ourselves with self-compassion gives us the resilience we need to take the risk of being vulnerable with each other in our relationships. True intimacy requires that we bring our true selves to our relationship. Without it we won't feel seen and loved. We can't possibly feel seen and loved when we are hiding ourselves and/or pretending to be something else so that others will like us.

Taking the time to develop our self-compassion practice benefits us both personally and relationally. Research shows people who have self-compassion have greater relationship satisfaction and a more secure attachment. They are more accepting of their partners and support the partner's autonomy while feeling more connected and less detached. Self-compassion is also associated with fewer controlling behaviors and less verbal and physical abuse. In the following chapters we will take a deeper dive into developing compassion for ourselves, our partners, and our relationships through the lens of the three components: mindfulness, common humanity, and self-kindness.

Part II

Building a Foundation for Compassion in Your Relationship

Mindfulness, Common Humanity, and Kindness

In this section, we move from understanding how things go awry in our relationships to cultivating the foundations of compassion for self and other through the lens of mindfulness, common humanity, and kindness. This section helps to open the heart and build (or strengthen) the solid bonds with each other based in kindness, caring, and compassion.

6

Being Present

Mindfulness Skills to See Clearly and Quiet Reactivity

Most people believe vulnerability is weakness. But really,
vulnerability is courage. We must ask ourselves . . . are we
willing to show up and be seen?

—BRENÉ BROWN

My first session with Hanna left me feeling a bit exhausted. For 50 minutes her anger at her partner blasted into every nook and cranny in my office as she detailed all of his character flaws. The most egregious of these flaws appeared to be that he never took her needs into account. That seemed to be at the root of her many stories of how she'd been overlooked and injured. She railed against his behavior. How could he just overlook her?! Everything in their lives seemed to revolve around his needs. I could see that she was angry and had been hurt. I wondered what that was like for her. What the effects of not having been seen and considered were for her. She had no interest in going there. She didn't want to talk about her own experience. She didn't want to talk about the fact that she was angry. When asked, she'd immediately head right back to detailing how he had wronged her. She was incensed and insisted that he needed to change.

This is a tricky situation for a therapist. It's like that old joke, "How many therapists does it take to change a lightbulb? One, but the lightbulb has to want to change." It's not uncommon for our patients to want us to change their parents, siblings, partners, children, colleagues, and others in their lives. Beyond the fact that we don't actually have the power to change other people, we can only work with those who are actually in the room. Hanna was here for individual therapy. Her partner had no interest in couples therapy. Beyond hearing her and validating that those situations would indeed be difficult to tolerate, continuing to discuss how her partner was a bad person in her eyes wasn't actually going to be helpful to Hanna. And she was determined that was exactly what we would be doing. What I knew she needed was to be seen. What she needed from her partner—to be seen and to matter—needed to happen in *our* session. I needed to see her and care about her so that she could begin to see and care about herself. What was exhausting about that first session was that her determination to focus on her partner was blocking Hanna from getting what she actually needed.

When our second session started out in just the same way, I knew I had to try something different. At some point I was able to say, "Your partner may indeed be all those things. I don't know; I haven't met him. But there is someone on the other side of things that is really hurting and yet isn't getting any attention—no attention from your partner and no attention from us either. And that person is you." She was stunned. There it was in full color. We were ignoring her too. Even here, in her private therapy session, her partner was getting all of the attention. The anger melded into sadness, and Hanna, at long last, entered the room for the first time.

We could now explore how awful it felt to want to be seen and to feel unseen, time and again. We looked at how unsafe that was for her. Her vulnerability was palpable. With anger, she had a protective shield that kept her from knowing and feeling what a vulnerable situation she was in. As we looked more deeply at her experience, she noticed how it was actually bigger than this one relationship. Most of her relationships were characterized by her focus on others to the exclusion of herself. In fact, the root of this seemed to be that as she grew up no one seemed to see or consider her. She could remember her father saying, "Children are to be seen and not heard." The way she learned to survive was to be alert to what others needed and behave in ways that were less likely to make her parents unhappy (and make her unsafe). This was indeed the best strategy for her in childhood. But in adulthood, this pattern kept her from seeing and tending to her own needs and left her vulnerable to being subsumed by others' wants and desires. She was so angry because she'd endured a lifetime of being marginalized.

Only by opening to and seeing her own experience was she going to be able to improve her situation. She had to start looking out for herself. She needed to move from her childhood position of longing to be seen by others so that *they* would tend to her needs and keep her safe into her own sense of agency. She needed to begin to be able to see herself so that *she* could tend to her needs and keep herself safe, even when others weren't able to do so for her. She needed to move from the question "Can *you* see me?" to the question "What is happening *for me* right now?"

Mindfulness along a Spectrum

The question "What is happening for me right now?" is actually the beginning of mindfulness, the first component of self-compassion. Neff's model emphasizes mindfulness versus overidentification. Overidentification, in this case, means rumination. Rumination occurs when we notice what is going on and become obsessed by it. Thoughts about it seemingly occupy our every waking moment, and we get stuck in the past (how bad it was) or the future (how bad it is going to be). We can create stories for ourselves, like my story about pain in my knee in the last chapter. When we get stuck in rumination, our vision is distorted. And our suffering increases.

I like to think about mindfulness, as well as the other two components of self-compassion, common humanity and self-kindness, as occurring on a spectrum, as the diagram on the next page shows.

Along the spectrum of mindfulness, if overidentification is on one end, at the other end of the spectrum we are unaware of our experience, as was Hanna. She was aware that she was angry, but just barely. Most of her attention was going to how bad her partner was. She actually spent very little time being curious about or understanding how she was feeling.

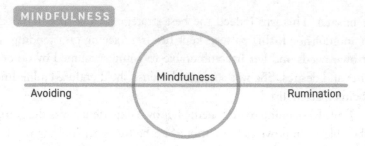

It makes sense, because she learned to survive her childhood of being unseen and unsafe by becoming somewhat invisible. She survived by not noticing her own pain. And now, when she did let herself know how painful it was for her, the pain felt unbearable. Initially, she felt powerless to change her situation, so not noticing was a kind of numbing for her. But this was really left over from her childhood, when she *was* powerless to change her situation. Now that she was an adult, she *had the power* to change her situation, although doing so would be difficult. What she needed was to claim that power through the clarity that comes when we open to and become curious about our own experience. Without being aware of the damage her marriage was doing to her, she would remain stuck and powerless to change it. In not seeing how *she* was feeling—a strategy from childhood to seek safety and avoid being in the threat/defense system—she was actually stuck in a relationship that chronically triggered her threat/defense system.

When Hanna began to open to and experience her anger, rather than just fixate on how bad her partner was, she began to get familiar with how anger felt in her own body. Her body got hot, her heart beat faster, and she was filled with energy. She could feel the power in the anger, and she was a little afraid of it too. Afraid that she would be destructive with her anger, as her parents sometimes had been with theirs. This realization was the beginning of Hanna's starting to reclaim a part of herself that had been forbidden.

Gradually she came to see that she could be empowered by her anger without acting in harmful ways. She also began to become aware of the pain underneath the anger. She could see the patterns of how she had felt powerless with her pain and how she'd developed a protective shield. That shield left her less vulnerable, but it also kept her from being seen and known in her primary relationship. Part of the reason her partner couldn't see her was that she kept herself hidden behind her shield to protect herself from being hurt. She didn't show her partner who she truly was. How could she when she herself didn't know?

> A shield can make us less vulnerable but also prevents us from being seen and known in our relationships.

The Power of Seeing Clearly

One aspect of mindfulness is the balanced awareness, or clear seeing, that comes when we open fully to our experience without pushing it away or exaggerating it. Of course, not noticing clouds our vision, and we don't see what is happening. But rumination also distorts our vision. Opening to things as they are, no more and no less, is empowering. When we are in touch with the truth of the situation, through our capacity to see clearly, we begin to understand what is needed. Knowledge is power. In Hanna's case, seeing more clearly allowed her to move from her stuck position into seeing herself and beginning to identify and honor her own needs and experiences. She also began healing from the pain she'd experienced earlier in her life—pain that left her with a crooked vision of things, the way the mirrors in the "fun house" distort our vision of reality. As she saw more clearly, she started to set limits with others and to tend to her own needs.

> Opening to things as they are, no more and no less, empowers us to see clearly and identify what is needed.

Not Seeing: A Strategy for Overwhelm

So why wouldn't we want to see? Well, often we resist and avoid what we don't like. It may feel painful or overwhelming to open fully to the truth of our situation. We may have tucked away our experience because we didn't have the resources to deal with it at the time. The good news is that this isn't an either/or situation. We can open fully to our situation, but we do so as we have the resources to manage the distress. Before "not noticing" was our (often unconscious) strategy to manage our distress. Now we can use other tools and skills to manage our distress, one powerful tool being the practice of mindfulness.

Mindfulness Practices to Restore Balance

Mindfulness is such a common label these days that it's hard to know what we really mean by the term. Jon Kabat-Zinn, who played a pivotal role in bringing mindfulness practice out of monasteries and into our ordinary lives, defines it as "the awareness that arises from paying attention, on purpose, in the present moment and nonjudgmentally." That definition, like all definitions, pales in comparison to the *experience* of mindfulness. It's akin to the difference between biting into a tasty peach at the peak of the season still warm from the sun and fresh off the tree and reading about what peaches taste like. Still, the medium we have here is words, so let's explore mindfulness as best we can, especially as it relates to our experience of relationships.

It is worth noting here that mindfulness is a topic that is much larger than we will have the time and space to explore fully. There is great value in developing a personal mindfulness practice. You'll find some resources for further exploration at the end of the book. For our purposes I'd like to focus here on ways that the practice of mindfulness can enhance relationships.

Two types of mindfulness practice can be especially helpful in developing skills that support the capacity for skillfully engaging in relationships. The first, concentrative awareness, can help us come into the moment in a way that stabilizes us. These are practices we can use to stay within or return to our window of tolerance (the place where we can still function even when feeling uncomfortable). The second type of practice, open monitoring, can help us expand our awareness and understanding of ourselves, our partners, and our relationships.

Concentrative Practices

Let's start by exploring concentrative awareness. When we are feeling unsafe or overwhelmed, concentrative awareness practices can help anchor us and help our physiology settle. Because threats to connection to our partners can feel life threatening, having practices to help anchor ourselves can help us stay or return to safely connecting. These practices can help us interrupt a downward relational spiral and change course.

In the beginning, as anger and its underlying fear arose for Hanna she often began to feel overwhelmed. When she did, we would stand together, shoulder to shoulder, as we looked at the tree outside my window. Hanna would describe the color and shape of the leaves, the texture of the bark, and so forth in great detail, and as she did her physiology would settle and she'd feel better. It was remarkably fast, often within only a minute or two. Hanna was using a concentrative awareness strategy by narrowly focusing her attention on the tree. Over time it became less scary for her to look at and be with the anger and underlying fear because she began to trust that she could find safety again simply by practicing looking deeply at things in nature.

We can actually choose where to place our attention. And different choices are likely to have different effects on us. Let's start by placing attention on an external object, as Hanna did.

TRY THIS

Noticing the Outer World

Take a moment now and bring your attention to something outside yourself, like a tree outside your window or a picture on the wall. Just for a few moments, let your attention rest on that one object.

Let yourself become more curious about this object, whether it is the first time you are seeing it or something you see all the time. Really look at it.

See the details. Looking at a tree, for example, notice the shape of the tree. Is it moving or still at the moment? How about the leaves or needles? Are there any? What shape and color are they? Do they clump together, or are they spread out? What about the branches? Is this a tree that grew straight and tall or one that spread out wide? How about the trunk of the tree? What is the texture? If you're up close to it, notice the smell and tactile sensation of the tree.

Let yourself be with the exploration of this object fully. Open to it with curiosity.

Stay with it as long as you like.

When your attention naturally ebbs, pause and notice how you feel.

What are the effects of this practice?

How are you feeling physically, emotionally, and mentally?

Now see if you want to continue to notice things. If you are done, perhaps thank yourself for paying attention to your life.

If you would like to continue, look around and see what else you'd like to be curious about. What else calls your attention?

Then, when something calls your attention, once again open with curiosity to that particular object.

Stay with it as long as you like, and when it feels like time to move on, you can choose another object or choose to close the practice for now.

Whenever you are done, please pause and notice any effects of your practice on you physically, mentally, or emotionally.

How do you feel now versus when you began?

In this practice we used concentrative awareness to focus on the object or string of objects that caught your attention. In between the objects, we used open awareness to see where your attention wanted to go. Most of us aren't aware that we have the power to shift our attention in this way and that this capacity to shift our attention from things and thoughts we find distressing to things we find safe and even pleasant can help us regulate our emotions. It can take us from feeling distressed to feeling calm, settled, and rooted. It doesn't make our problems go away, of course, but it does help us dial back the overwhelming feelings. Focusing on things outside ourselves allows our physiology to settle. Practicing this over and over can give us the confidence and resources to begin to open more fully to our situation, because we know how to settle and calm when life feels overwhelming.

Another anchor for awareness that you might experiment with is noticing where your body is making contact with something outside your body. For example, where is your body making contact with the chair, bed, floor, or earth right now? Can you feel the pressure and other sensations where the body is making contact? Is there warmth, for example? What about where your body is making contact with your clothes? Stay here as long as you like, perhaps even as little as one or two minutes. Then notice the impact of paying attention in this way. One of my favorite activities is paying attention to the soles of the feet as they make contact with the ground. Perhaps you'd like to try it too?

TRY THIS
Soles of the Feet

Audio Track 10

It helps, if possible, to stand so that the sensation of the feet making contact with the ground is easier to feel. However, if standing is difficult for you for any reason, this practice can also be done while sitting.

Allow your attention to settle, like silt in a lake, all the way down to the sensations on the very bottom of your feet. What do you notice here?

It can also help to slowly circle the knees around in one direction and then the other, creating changing sensations in the soles of the feet, or to lean left, right, forward, back. Notice areas of pressure, of no contact, warmth, moisture—whatever is there.

We can also take these feet on a little walk, by taking slow and gentle steps, one at a time, noticing the changing sensations on the soles of the feet. Perhaps there are now different sensations as the foot flexes, the heel lands, and the pressure rolls to the balls of the feet.

The mind may wander back to your problems, but that is no problem. Just gently and firmly return your attention to the sensations of the soles of the feet.

When you feel done, take some time to notice the effects of this exercise.

You might notice that it is easier for you to focus your attention while you are still. Or it may be easier for you to focus your attention while you are moving. There is no right or wrong here, just whatever works best for you. And at different times you may prefer one or the other. For example, when you are sad you may like to be still, and when you are anxious you may prefer movement. The more you experiment with practices, the more you will discover what works best for you. You will develop a toolbox you can open when you become distressed.

Another possibility, and another favorite of mine, is to anchor your awareness on a bodily function, especially the breath. You might like to experiment with this, too.

TRY THIS
Awareness of Breath

Audio Track 11

Start in a comfortable position that also enables you to stay alert. Sitting with a straight (but not rigid) back is often helpful here, but do find whatever position gives you a sense of relaxation along with alertness.

When you're ready, you might like to close your eyes if it makes it easier to focus inwardly.

As you bring your attention inside the body, become curious about the sensation of breathing in the body.

- You can start to label and notice "inhale" and "exhale," for example, becoming ever more curious about what it feels like to inhale and what it feels like to exhale.

- You can keep your focus on a particular area of the body, such as the edge of the nostrils, the rising and falling of the chest, or the expanding and contracting of the belly.
- Or you can focus more broadly on the sensation of the whole body breathing in and breathing out.

You might begin to notice how the body is nourished on the inhale. The oxygen flows in with the breath and eventually is distributed throughout the body, nourishing the whole body. And how the body releases what it no longer needs through the exhale, relaxing and releasing. Take some time to feel into that now if you like.

After a while, begin to notice the rhythm of the breath. Like waves in the ocean, the breath flows in and out. Perhaps even notice if there is a subtle rocking of the body as the ribcage expands and contracts. Rest in the gentle, rhythmic flow of the breath.

Whenever you feel ready, let go of the particular focus on the breath and just rest inside your body and notice any effects of this practice.

For many, the breath can become a soothing anchor—one that is portable. We take it with us wherever we go, and we don't even need to close our eyes to tune in to the breath. We can do it in any situation, and no one even needs to know. For others, however, it may not feel right. I had severe pneumonia as a teenager and have some scarring in my lung. Although the breath has indeed become a place of refuge for me, it wasn't this way in the beginning. I had to go slowly with it, not pushing myself to continue if it activated my threat/defense system. I moved into the practice when it felt safe for me and chose one of the other mindfulness practices when it began to feel overwhelming. You'll need to use your own judgment about which practices feel helpful and when to use them too.

Finding the right practice for you may involve some experimenting. My hope is that throughout this book you'll experiment to find what works best for you and end up with something that is customized for you.

Concentrative Practices Can Restore Safety

There is an optimal amount of arousal when learning new things. Teachers today use Dan Siegel's term for this: the *window of tolerance*. Some of us shut down when we become stressed, and others of us feel overwhelmed. We don't learn much when we are hypo- or hyper-aroused. We want to stay in the zone that allows us to open safely. Much like the mindfulness spectrum, we want to stay in—or, more accurately, return to, again and again—the balanced awareness part of the spectrum. Out of avoidance or not noticing and out of rumination and overwhelm. Using mindfulness practices can help us find our way back to the window of tolerance whenever we find ourselves shutting down or overwhelmed. Often people find that the farther away from the body they place their attention, the safer they feel. If you find yourself outside your window of tolerance when following your breath, you may find Soles of the Feet or Noticing the Outer World restores a sense of safety. Now that you have these mindfulness skills, it may be easier to go back and try any self-reflection exercises you skipped in Part I of the book. You can center and ground yourself any time you feel the need.

Open Monitoring: Mindfulness Practices to Help Us See Clearly

In his definition of mindfulness Kabat-Zinn notes that we are paying attention *on purpose, in the present moment*. For most of us, this means that mindfulness starts with having the intention of paying attention to this moment. To continue our earlier peach analogy, how many times have you eaten something without really tasting it? Maybe you were distracted by work, or by the person you were talking to, or maybe by thoughts from the past or worries about the future. When, however, we decide that there is benefit in paying attention to something like the peach, and we set our intention to notice our experience of eating the peach, we become aware of the taste, texture, juiciness, temperature, smell of the peach, and we have a more full experience of the peach.

How much attention do you pay to your own experiences day to day? Do you notice what is happening in your body moment to moment—a feeling of ease, tightness in the shoulders, an achiness in the chest, or clenching of the belly? Are you aware of which emotions are present? Which thoughts you are having and whether they are a pattern for you? Many of us live on autopilot, skimming the surface of our lives.

How much attention do you pay to your partner's experience day to day? Are you present on purpose or kinda checked out—skimming the surface, waiting for clues you should tune in?

Most of us go through life in a kind of autopilot way, unless something highly positive or highly negative grabs our attention. This may be our default, but we can reset the default. It starts with the intention to pay attention to the present moment—and to the people in the present moment.

In terms of setting an intention to show up and pay attention to yourself, your partner, and your relationship, you're already off to a great start. You're reading this book. In terms of paying attention, open monitoring practices have us opening fully to whatever arises while we pay attention in the moment.

Just as we use concentrative practice to feel safe, we can use open monitoring practices to deepen our understanding and grow wiser. This practice helps us see things we haven't previously noticed.

In open monitoring practice, we are already feeling anchored and rooted and we open our awareness to notice and experience whatever arises. We try to stay on the noticing side, not getting caught liking or not liking and not pushing experiences away or trying to hold on to pleasant experiences. We practice noticing what is here without trying to control it. Curiosity and nonjudgment are helpful attitudes. One way to practice this is to open to sound.

TRY THIS

Awareness of Sound

Audio Track 12

Find a comfortable position for yourself, then set a timer. It could be for 3 minutes, 30 minutes, or anything in between.

After settling into the moment and the body, open to sounds as they arise.

You might first notice sounds (or a lack thereof) that are happening outside the room—perhaps the call of a bird, a jack-hammer, the sound of a horn, or ocean waves crashing.

As best you can, let go of whether you find the sound pleasant or unpleasant. Let go of needing to label it. Just receive sounds as they arise and as they vibrate your eardrums, resting in the experience of sounds.

Now expand your awareness to include sounds inside your room. In the same way, open to and receive whatever arises, including silence.

Finally, expand your awareness even further, this time including sounds that arise from inside your body as well. Perhaps notice gurgles in the stomach or the sound of your heart beating.

Again opening with curiosity, see what arises and let sounds come and go without the added dimension of liking or not liking.

This is like a private symphony that will never come again. Open to and receive whatever arises.

Were you able to open to sounds as they arose without getting carried away by thoughts or by liking or not liking? Did you discover things you might have missed if you hadn't intentionally tuned in to sounds around you? Most of us do find we discover new things when we practice open monitoring meditation. Perhaps you noticed that we have a choice about how broadly we open our attention? When we limited the focus to sounds outside the room, were you also aware of sounds inside your body?

This practice can be done with anything. We can use any of our five senses to notice the world: sight, smell, taste, touch, or sound. And we can use these five senses (or sense doors) to identify what is happening with people too. An angry red face or a loud and sharp voice comes in through our sight and sound senses, and we understand our partners are angry, for example. In open monitoring we use our skills to open with curiosity to the world around and within us.

Open Monitoring Can Help Us Learn and Grow

When we are closed down, as in hypoarousal and not noticing, open monitoring can help us open again and find our way back into the window of tolerance, where we are more likely to learn and grow. Likewise, we can use open monitoring to become aware of our relational patterns. We can shift our attention to our partners and what is happening with them. We can shift our attention to ourselves and what is happening within us. And we can also shift our attention to see the relational patterns of how we interact with each other. We see how our own tendency to get defensive, critical, or controlling gets in the way of safety for our partners, ourselves, and our relationships. As we explored in Part I of this book, we see how, like the porcupine with its quills out, we are actually getting in the way of what we want in our relationships. And when we see our patterns more clearly, we often begin to see the path forward more clearly.

Attitude Is Everything

When someone pays attention to us, *how* they pay attention is everything. Ever talk with someone who seemed like judge and jury and was waiting to tell you everything you did wrong? I bet you didn't want to go to them with your difficulties, knowing you would be met with that attitude. It tends to shut one down. That's why in Kabat-Zinn's definition of mindfulness he notes that it requires nonjudgment. Whether we are exploring our own experience, that of our partner, or our relational patterns, nonjudgment is essential.

Nonjudgment

In opening to what is, it is helpful to approach with a nonjudgmental attitude of friendliness. When we remember this is someone we care about—not an enemy even if the person has done something harmful, but simply a person who has behaved unskillfully—we can stay present and out of judgment. It helps to remember how human it is to behave unskillfully and make mistakes. What Brené Brown refers to as generosity is part of this attitude. Generosity in this context means assuming the best in ourselves and our partners. Most often the unskillful action that hurts one partner is rooted in the pain and misunderstanding of the other. And our own pain and misunderstanding of *their* action usually leads to our own unskillful behavior—and a downward relational spiral.

Curiosity

Rather than judgment, bringing an attitude of curiosity is essential. Wanting to know and understand helps open our minds and hearts. We can have a sense of curiosity about our own behavior ("I wonder why I was so quick to anger; was there some hurt underneath?") and about our partner's ("I wonder why he was so quick to anger; was there hurt or fear underneath?"). This allows our understanding to reach beneath the surface and allows us to address what our partner needs from a place of wisdom rather than reactivity. We begin to see patterns over time, and we understand what would be skillful. The attitude of curiosity also softens us, and we can approach our partners from a more receptive and vulnerable place, which increases safety for our partners and leads to their being much more likely to soften with us as well.

Acceptance

Acceptance really is at the heart of what we want from each other, isn't it? When we can bring ourselves to be vulnerable enough to be truly seen, and we are accepted as we are, we feel loved. It can be challenging to accept imperfections in our partners and relationships, but when we truly understand that being imperfect is part of the shared human condition, we can begin to know ourselves, our partners, and our relationships as perfectly imperfect.

Acceptance doesn't mean that we are saying we are okay with things that need to change. We still need limits and boundaries. It simply means that we are opening to the truth that this is how things are right now. Allowing—accepting the truth of what is—makes it possible for a deeper wisdom to arise. As first mentioned in Chapter 3, psychologist Carl Rogers said, "The curious paradox is that when I accept myself as I am, then I can change." Acceptance works that way with partners too.

Mindfulness in Three Directions

Mindfulness then, has two important qualities for us. It helps us see more clearly, leading to wise choices. It also helps us find and return to safety when we inevitably become triggered, so that we can act out of responsiveness rather than reactivity. Over time, it helps us change our relational patterns into ones that foster good healthy relationships.

> Mindfulness helps us see clearly enough to make wise choices and also to return to safety when triggered. The result is responsiveness instead of reactivity in our relationships.

When we toggle back and forth this way, opening to the painful truth of our situation and then, if we begin to feel overwhelmed, narrowing our focus to a safe object, we begin to *safely* open to the truth of our experience and our situation, as we are ready to do so. This sense of safety gives us a new confidence that we can indeed be with what we need to be with. We can begin to see and understand ourselves. When we can trust our capacity to return to safety, we can begin to become more comfortable with our vulnerability. We can even begin to let our partners see who we truly are—fears, wounds, and all. And that willingness to be seen forms the basis for true intimacy.

Seeing Ourselves

When we open with curiosity and acceptance to our own experience, we also move from focusing on needing our *partners* to see us to seeing *ourselves*, moving out of the dependent state we were in as children and into the empowered state of adulthood. We can see ourselves now, and ultimately that leads to having the courage to allow ourselves to *be seen*, to *make ourselves visible* to our partners. Allowing ourselves to be seen lays the foundation for true intimacy in our relationships.

For Hanna, learning to see herself and knowing how to return to safety gave her the courage to let her partner know what was truly happening for her. Where before she would angrily blast her partner for not considering her needs, she was now able to calmly let him know that she didn't feel like being intimate with him, for example, because she didn't feel seen when he committed them to going to his parents' house without checking to be sure it was okay with her first—especially since she'd expressed how difficult this was for her many times. And she was able to ask for what she needed—could he just make a habit of letting his parents know he needed to check with her first to be sure?

In Part I there were a lot of self-reflection prompts to help you begin to uncover your own personal relational patterns. I hope you were able to bring the intentions of wisdom and compassion to the reflections, and the attitudes of nonjudgment, curiosity, and acceptance toward yourself, as you began to look more deeply into the ways in which you tend to operate when you feel threatened (blame, withdraw, placate), when you are attempting to get out of pain by some form of resistance (usually involving the drive system: fix, control, criticize), and when you feel cared about. Opening to and seeing our relational patterns is mindfulness in action.

Over time, when we practice open monitoring, we begin to notice patterns in what we feel and how we relate to others. Heart pounding and fullness in the head may happen alongside the emotion of anger, for example. And these feelings may precede blaming others. Or feeling shaky or a knot in the stomach may come alongside fear, which may precede checking out of a relationship. And you can notice that that is a familiar feeling that reminds you of when you were little and your dad was angry and you felt unsafe and powerless, to continue the example. Your experience of these things may vary. My point is that we begin to identify our own personal relational patterns, how these patterns may result from earlier experiences, and the cues that one of our patterns has been activated. When we can identify that one of our patterns is activated, and we pause to allow our physiology to recover (often with concentrative awareness practices), we have the power to choose a different response. Opening to our own experiences with curiosity, acceptance, and nonjudgment allows us to see clearly and to make choices based in wisdom. Though we can sometimes be frightened to allow ourselves to know the truth of things, when we do we have the power to choose our response. In that choice lies our freedom and our growth.

A practice I like for this is the STOP practice. This practice has been circulating in mindfulness circles for some time. Here is my take on how this practice can be helpful.

TRY THIS
STOP

Audio Track 13

Please find a comfortable position and allow your eyes to close, or take a soft gaze toward the floor.

If it feels right, perhaps place a hand on your heart, or anywhere else that might feel supportive as a way of reminding yourself of the intention to pay kind attention to yourself as you go through this exercise.

Now call to mind some sort of difficulty that you are in the midst of right now. This could be a relational issue, or it could be something else. It could be feeling stressed about something at work, or something with a family member, or perhaps it is a health issue. Something that generates a little stress in your body but isn't overwhelming. A 3–4 on the distress scale of 1–10, where 1 is no stress and 10 is extremely stressful.

Let yourself visualize this situation or just open to the felt sense of the situation.

And now, as best you can, STOP:

S—Stop. Let go of the story line. Pause and open to this moment here.

T—Take a breath. Turn your attention toward your breathing. Notice where you feel the breath most easily in the body, or perhaps notice the rhythm of the breath. If the breath isn't a safe anchor for you, please choose something else to concentrate on, like the soles of the feet.

O—Observe. Now see if you can expand your perspective of the situation. With curiosity, ask yourself, "What is really going on here?" "What am I missing?" Open to more information about yourself and/or others in the situation.

Ask yourself, given all of this, "What do I need right now? Perhaps a soothing touch? Some kind words of understanding and reassurance? A self-compassion break? A form of behavioral self-compassion, like pausing for a cup of tea or taking a short walk?"

P—Proceed to practice. As best you can, give yourself whatever you need at this moment.

Whenever we find ourselves triggered and unlikely to interact skillfully with our partners, taking a moment to tend to ourselves with practices like the STOP practice can be really wise. We want to tend to our own physiology first so that we have the capacity to engage with our partners skillfully.

Seeing Our Partners

In this chapter we have explored mindfulness skills that you can use to center and calm yourself when you are outside your window of tolerance (concentrative skills: Noticing the Outer World, Soles of the Feet, and Awareness of Breath), and also to open to what is around and within you with curiosity and acceptance (open monitoring skills: Awareness of Sound). We can use the same skills when we want to truly see our partners.

We have spent quite a lot of time in reflection exercises to see our partners more clearly in Part I, so you may already be aware of your partner's patterns and tender spots. It can also be helpful to learn how to see your partner in the present moment. It is often easier to develop a skill when we are not distressed, so the following practice begins this way. (Later we will introduce a practice to see your partner when you—and your partner—are distressed.) This practice is a good one to lay the foundation for seeing our partners in the present moment. Let's try that now (or later if your partner isn't around right now).

TRY THIS
Seeing Your Partner

At a time when your partner is present, set your intention to pay attention to them with the attitudes of curiosity, nonjudgment, and acceptance.

If you are not interacting, begin by looking at your partner (as unobtrusively as possible).

What do you see? What does your partner's body look like? Is there hair? What color is it? Is it long or short, curly or straight? See if you can become curious about what your partner actually looks like.

Notice if feelings of liking or not liking arise in you and recognize that is judgment.

See if you can go back to seeing your partner as your partner is and accepting the truth of how they look in this moment.

Notice also if your partner's body looks comfortable or if there are signs that discomfort or pain is present. What is your sense of your partner's physical state?

There are other clues in the body too. Clues that can give you some idea about the emotional state your partner is in.

- Is your partner smiling?
- Does the face look peaceful, tired, sleepy?
- Is the face looking sad, angry, scared?
- What about the rest of the body?
- If you were a detective, what would you imagine your partner's emotional state is right now?

If you are interacting, add in the aspect of listening to them.

- What is your partner actually saying?
- What does your partner want you to know?
- What is their perspective?
- Do you get a sense of their mental state?

Given your observations, do you have a sense of whether your partner is in distress at the moment? If so, are there any clues to what your partner might want or need from you?

If a desire to offer your partner comfort or other types of support arises, know that this is a theory you have about them—informed by your observations. You can check out your theory by offering your partner the support. Be sure to make a mental note about whether your partner actually wanted the support you offered, especially if there is something else they needed.

What happened when you took the time and intentionally placed your attention on seeing your partner? Did you learn anything? It's not uncommon that a feeling of closeness arises just from seeing your partner.

Seeing Our Relationship Interaction Patterns

When we can bring this attitude of curiosity without judgment to ourselves and our partners, it becomes possible to see how our tendencies interact with each other. In other words, we can become aware of our relationship interaction patterns. We see, for example, how the more we withdraw the harder our partners try to gain our attention (pursue) or how the more we pursue our partners the harder our partners try to get away and get some space (withdraw).

In Part I you may have become more familiar with how relationship interaction patterns play out in your own relationship. In the Compassion for Couples program we have a simple exercise that helps to give a felt sense to the conceptual understanding. It's an exercise that partners do together, but if your partner isn't willing to do it with you, you can do it with a friend. You will still get a felt sense. Here is how it goes:

Touching Hands

Audio Track 14

Stand (or sit) facing one another. Now both partners hold up one palm. It should be one person's left and the other's right palm so that they are mirror images.

Now bring your hands together, palm to palm.

Okay, now try that again. This time, bring them together slowly while paying attention to the sensations in your hand as you bring your hand slowly closer, and eventually touch your partner's hand.

Okay, this time, bring them together again slowly, while focusing on your partner's hand.

Then rest here with hands touching for a moment and notice what it is like to be both present and connected in this way.

Often something happens; perhaps we get scared and withdraw. The person with the longer first name, please quickly withdraw your hand. Notice what it felt like to withdraw your hand or what it felt like for your partner to withdraw their hand.

Please bring your hands together again, and the second partner quickly withdraw your hand when you are ready. Notice what it felt like to withdraw your hand or what it felt like for your partner to withdraw their hand.

This is what distancing feels like. Notice which was a more familiar feeling—withdrawing or being left. Also notice what it felt like to be on the other side of what you usually do.

And bringing the hands back together again, the person with the longer name now straighten your arm and push your hand into your partner's hand. Once again noticing what it felt like to be the person who pushed, or the person who was pushed. This is what it feels like when one person pursues.

Now bring the hands back together so the other partner can push their hand into their partner's hand. Again noting what it felt like to be pursued or to pursue.

Notice which was a more familiar feeling—pursuing or being pursued. Also notice what it felt like to be on the other side of what you usually do.

And bringing the hands together one last time, see if you might move the hands around together. "Dancing" together. No need to keep the palms together all the time, just noting how they relate to each other.

What did you discover about your own pattern and how it may feel for your partner to be on the other side of it? When we do this exercise in class, often people who withdraw are stunned by the pain they feel when their partner withdraws their hand suddenly. And feeling this pain begins to give people a sense of what it feels like for their partners when they disappear, which often motivates them to try a new pattern. Instead of just disappearing, they can still take space. But first they reassure their partners that they are loved and they are coming back, by saying something like "I'm really charged up right now. I'm gonna take some time and see if I can settle down a bit. I still care about you and our relationship. Can we try this conversation again after lunch?"

On the other end of things, you may have identified as having a pattern of pursuing. What did it feel like when your partner pushed their hand into yours? Did it feel intrusive? Most often it does for people. How did you respond to this intrusion? Did you collapse your own arm? Did you push back? What did your partner do? People often get to experience what it is like to be on the receiving end of their personal strategies for restoring safety. We can see that these tend to dance together—people who feel intruded upon (pursued) tend to withdraw. People who feel abandoned (when their partners suddenly withdraw) tend to pursue to keep a connection going. And we can see how these strategies are creating a larger relationship interaction pattern that isn't working. The funny thing is that just the awareness itself of these relationship interaction patterns often provides enough wisdom and motivation for one or both partners to begin to change the pattern by shifting their own behavior.

We can also place our attention on that feeling of being connected. What might happen if you noticed the ways in which you do feel connected more often? Here is a short practice inspired by the renowned teacher Thich Nhat Hanh:

TRY THIS

Feeling Connected

When you are naturally feeling connected to your partner, or it feels natural to stand by them, hold their hand, or give them a hug, for example, take a moment to notice each of these three things briefly:

- I am alive
- My partner is here
- How precious it is that we are together (connected)

Once again you can notice how it feels after this brief practice. Practicing noticing how it feels to be connected can begin to shift us into the affiliation of the care system where we feel safe, connected, and content.

Practicing mindfulness can help us find our way back to safety when we feel overwhelmed, and it can help us see ourselves, our partners, and our relationships more clearly. We begin to see and understand which patterns create downward spirals in our relationships and how we can interrupt the spiral and settle our own physiology, see our partners, and choose a wise response. Best of all, it helps us see into the nature of being a human being. We see that when we are unskillful in how we relate to our partner it isn't some diabolical intention, or a sign that we don't care about our partners—rather it is an attempt to keep ourselves safe. The same is true for our partners. And when we can stop taking their behavior personally, combined with beginning to take personal responsibility for our own behavior and needs, often a downward spiral turns instead to an upward spiral. We will explore this ability to see into the nature of being human more fully in the next chapter.

7

Cultivating Connection

Strength in Common Humanity

If we have no peace, it is because we have forgotten that we
belong to each other.

—MOTHER TERESA

By definition being in a relationship means there is some sort of connection between two people, and that is important because we are
wired to belong. Belonging is so important that we are acutely aware
of not feeling like we belong and what we think will keep us from
belonging. We also give up ourselves in an effort to belong. Sometimes
we focus so much on what we think others want from us, we don't
even know what we ourselves want. We lose touch with ourselves in
the pursuit of being connected. But when we don't bring our true self
into the relationship, the relationship becomes a mere structure, one
that lacks a soul. Both people have to be fully human and present to
belong. It's like the difference between a house and a home.

This is a tender topic for us; belonging is so core to our sense of
survival. And it is this very desire for belonging that is at the root of so
much of the pain in our relationships. Belonging and mattering to
someone else is most salient when it comes to common humanity—the
second component of self-compassion. Neff describes it as common
humanity versus isolation. She points out that when things go wrong
for us, we tend to think everyone else is doing well and we alone are
struggling. This was the case for my friend Valerie in Chapter 2. She
thought she was the only one who was in the midst of the pain of living

with an addict. Of course, logically she knew that she wasn't the only one. It's just that when she looked around at her friends and neighbors she didn't see anyone else with problems. Well, when she let herself really look, she had to admit that some of her friends had problems. But, she was quick to add, their problems looked small in comparison.

> A relationship without both partners fully present and human is just a structure—a house but not a home.

Isolation: It's All about Me

As Neff notes, Valerie felt isolated. She felt all alone with her problems. And she felt something else—shame. She couldn't understand why her husband wasn't satisfied with their life together. They had all the trappings: two kids, a nice home, and even a dog. She didn't really know what the problem was. What was so wrong with their life that he needed to numb himself? The only thing she could think of was that the problem was her. It must be her. There must be something wrong with her. She'd grown up in a family that was struggling to make ends meet, and he'd grown up in a very affluent family. His family, especially his mother, had made it clear that Valerie wasn't cultured enough for them. She was always trying to be good enough for her mother-in-law. In fact, all her life she'd been trying to be good enough and had fallen short in someone else's eyes. Things were hard in her current family. It seemed that she didn't really matter. If only she were good enough, maybe she would matter too, she thought.

Why Don't I Belong?

As a therapist who has worked with children, I know that when things go wrong in their lives, whether it is something big or a series of smaller things, the most common reaction they have is to believe there is something wrong with them. It would be unfathomable for a vulnerable child to know that bad things can happen at any time and that they are powerless to do anything about it. So sewn into the lining of that story is hope—the hope that if there is indeed something bad about them that caused the problem, then if they change maybe bad things will stop happening. It's a child's way of inventing power when they don't have any.

That's what happened for Valerie. As she was growing up things were hard. She didn't feel safely connected, and the more she longed to belong, the more alone and rejected she felt. The kids at school teased her. They felt her desperation to belong, and they felt more powerful when they teased her. It's not that she deserved to be teased in any way. It's that they themselves felt insecure and somehow they felt more secure about their own belonging when they banded together in putting her down.

It's not hard to understand why Valerie thought there was something wrong with her. Her whole life she'd been given that message—first at home, then with her peers, then by her mother-in-law, and eventually by her husband too. However, that never was the truth then and it wasn't the truth now. Of course she had her oddities and rough edges. All of us have our own oddities and rough edges to varying degrees. Those things made her unique, but they didn't make her unlovable or undeserving of belonging.

Sometimes It's Just a Mismatch

Feeling like we don't belong isn't always a result of having oddities and rough edges. Often it is more a matter of having talents and values that differ from the values in our families and communities. For example, maybe you are creative and artistic, but you grew up in a family that saw little value in creative pursuits. Your family placed greater value on being smart and achieving financial success. Of course it is equally possible that you were naturally smart and driven toward achievement and financial success, but you grew up in a family that valued art and creativity. Either scenario would naturally lead you to feel there was something wrong with you. Even if you were both smart and artistically inclined you might come away feeling there was something wrong with the part of you that valued what your family didn't see value in.

Maybe it's more a question of temperament. Perhaps you identify as more introverted and your family lived a more extroverted lifestyle. Or the other way round. Or maybe you were born to explore and are always keen for the next adventure, and you grew up in a small town. There are endless examples of possible mismatches. The point is that it is easy to feel like there is something wrong with you when it's really just a mismatch. One common clue to this is feeling like you are "not enough" or "too much."

Jean Shinoda Bolen, Jungian analyst and expert in Greek mythology, tells the myth of the procrustean bed in her book *Gods in Everyman* to illustrate what happens to us when there is a mismatch. In ancient Greece, as the story goes, all travelers on their way to Athens would meet up with Procrustes and his bed. Before being allowed to proceed they would be placed on his bed, and anyone who was too short would be stretched to fit the bed, as if on a medieval torture rack. Anything that hung over the bed would be lopped off. She explains that in ancient times Athens was the center of things and anyone who wanted to belong would need to travel there. The journey to belonging required conformity.

Growing up in a financially oriented family when you are an artist often translates to having your creativity lopped off and your financial acumen stretched to fit. Similarly, growing up in an artistic family when you are financially oriented would require having your financial acumen lopped off (or cut down to size) and your artistic talents stretched to fit. Of course, hard as we may try to conform by stretching and lopping off, we are aware that we just don't fit.

As we feel that lack of belonging, we don't understand it is a mismatch. We can't see the bigger picture well enough. We believe the story that there is something wrong with us that makes us unworthy of belonging. We believe that we're unworthy of anyone's time and attention—never mind their love and affection.

Common Humanity: Everyone Belongs

Believing we're unworthy of love and affection causes us to show up in our relationships as if we don't matter. We send the message to our partners that our needs are unimportant in the relationship, and then we feel upset when the relationship revolves around the other person. Feeling unworthy is also a problem when we then try to practice self-compassion, in particular common humanity. Common humanity by its definition says everyone belongs. We are part of this shared human condition with its beauty and joys and also with its sorrows and shortcomings.

Common humanity isn't *sameness*. It doesn't say that we all have the same degree of joy or struggle, for example. Some of us suffer much more than others of us ever could fathom—especially those who are marginalized and oppressed in our culture. Common humanity is about *belonging and mattering*. It says we all belong to the human species, no matter our shape, color, ability, gender identification or sexual orientation, or whatever our particular identities might be. Every last one of us belongs. And it says that by virtue of belonging, each of us matters.

This belonging means that when we feel isolated, and believe there is something wrong with us, that we don't matter, as Valerie did, we are not seeing clearly. Yes, we may have been marginalized in our family of origin, in our primary relationship, or in our society. *But being marginalized can never take away the fact that you are part of the shared human condition.* While society may value some more than others, that is an error on the part of the people who seek power by marginalizing others. It is never an accurate reflection of your true value. The most tragic part of being marginalized, though, is that when we internalize this devaluing we don't treat ourselves with an appreciation of our own worth and we act in our relationships and our lives as if our own suffering doesn't matter.

> When we internalize being devalued by society, we act—in our relationships and the rest of life—as if our own pain doesn't matter.

To be human means to experience the hardships of life and to have struggles in our relationships. When we understand that others are suffering too—others whose relationships are strained to the point of breaking, or have a family member whose addiction is causing distress in the family, who have the same identities we have and have also been marginalized, who feel like there is something wrong with them and think they just don't matter—and we open our heart to their suffering, then we can, perhaps, include ourselves in our kind wishes for relief of suffering. Without a firm grasp on this belonging and shared human condition, when we fall into the illusion of isolation, any kindness we offer ourselves is likely to be tinged with pity. Unlike compassion, pity says we are somehow less than others. This misconception can keep us feeling separate from others. When we broaden our vision to include the truth that others struggle and suffer too, we activate the affiliative system, which leads to activation of the care system. We are not alone. We begin to discover that we matter and belong—even if the particular relationship we are in doesn't reflect our value.

> When we understand that others struggle too, we activate the care system—and suddenly we are no longer alone.

TRY THIS
Discovering Common Humanity

Audio Track 15

Reflect for a moment on one of the ways in which you feel you are falling short or suffering in ways that others don't understand. For example, maybe you got fired from your job and you don't know anyone else who's been fired. Or perhaps your boss just told you that you need to improve in something. Or maybe your partner has let you know that you are falling short. Maybe your partner has even left you or threatened to leave. Maybe you have a health problem or something that makes you feel less physically attractive to others. Maybe you've been marginalized by society for the color of your skin, your gender or sexual orientation, or your religion, for example.

Take a moment now and acknowledge that thing that makes you feel isolated, alone, or unlovable.

Can you give it a name?

Now consider whether any of your friends or family have experienced something similar. For example, if you feel unattractive, is there anyone else in your circle of family or friends who isn't known for being attractive? Might they have struggled with feeling unattractive too? It's quite common not to meet society's expectations of attractiveness, with its retouched photos and narrow definition of beauty. If so, notice what arises in you in terms of acceptance and kindness when you think about the situation they were or are in.

Now, broadening your circle of compassion to include acquaintances, have any of them experienced something similar, even if it was more or less pronounced? If so, notice what you have said or would say to them if you bumped into them and the subject came up. Would you give them the benefit of the doubt? Would you offer them kindness and understanding?

Now, broadening your circle of compassion even further to include people you don't know—everyone in your neighborhood, city, state, country, and even the world—can you imagine, even though you don't know them, how many others share your situation right this minute?

Picturing or having a felt sense of all of you together, would they be surprised to discover they are not alone? Are you surprised to discover you are not alone? What does it feel like to know you are not alone?

What kind wishes or words of encouragement do you have for them? Can you include yourself in that circle of compassion? Can you offer yourself the kindness you need?

Take a moment and notice the effects of recognizing that you are not alone and offering kindness to yourself and others.

Common Humanity: The Full Spectrum

As I mentioned in Chapter 6, I see each of the three components of self-compassion along a spectrum. With common humanity, isolation or "it's just me" does live on one end of the spectrum. On the other end of the spectrum we think "it's just them." We think, "Others have it worse than I do, so my struggles and suffering don't matter. I should be giving all of my compassion to others because they have it worse than I do." Common humanity, however, sits in the middle of the spectrum, as shown in the diagram below. It says "everyone matters" and "everyone belongs." True, at any given moment it might be skillful to focus more on ourselves or more on another, based on the degree of suffering in this moment. In the end, though, we have a responsibility to include everyone in our circle of compassion.

It's All about Others—I Don't Matter

I was surprised the first time "it's just them" showed up in a class I was teaching on mindful self-compassion. The participant clearly had been through a lot and was suffering, but her practice of self-compassion seemed to be blocked by something. When I inquired further, she explained that she felt guilty offering herself compassion for what she saw as a little thing compared to the real suffering that others were experiencing. She thought that all of her attention and goodwill should go to those who were suffering more than she was, even though her suffering *was* causing significant issues for her. This was the crux of why she'd come to this course. She knew she needed self-compassion like one needs a drop of water in the desert. She was parched. And yet she was stuck believing that she couldn't have any as long as others were suffering more than she was.

The irony is that she was in a five-day intensive workshop to learn self-compassion. There was nothing she could do in this moment to benefit others (except that self-compassion does benefit others, and

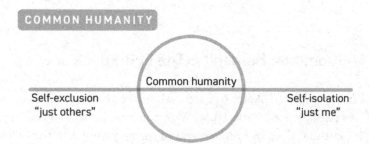

we'll explore that more in a bit). We explored whether withholding compassion for herself was benefiting others. She couldn't really say it was, even though she was sure it worked that way. It's the kind of answer that arises when we have bought into a core belief that isn't actually based in fact. So I asked her what she would say to me if I had the same pain as she had, but my co-teacher had a worse situation. Did she think I should I deny myself compassion because my colleague had a worse situation? She was horrified. "Of course not!" she was quick to say. And she began to see that we are all worthy of compassion, regardless of whether our suffering is big or small in any particular moment.

Triage of Compassion—Who Needs What When

This idea that others are more important is something I see in just about every class I teach. The confusion usually boils down to timing. Sometimes the practice of compassion is like triage—we tend to the most wounded first. This is often true in the initial stages of couples therapy. When both partners are suffering on multiple levels, we do need to tend to the most vulnerable first. For example, if someone is suicidal and the other is anxious, the suicidal person will get my attention first—in the same way that someone who is having a heart attack would get medical attention before someone with indigestion. Eventually, though, even that person with chronic indigestion would need attention. It isn't a matter of saying "I only have indigestion and there are people out there having heart attacks, so don't worry about me." With self-compassion, this strategy breaks down even further. It boils down to "I'm going to ignore my indigestion because people in the world are having heart attacks." Sounds kind of crazy when I put it that way, doesn't it? We have a responsibility to take care of ourselves. When we include ourselves in our circle of compassion, we are better able to care for others.

The More I Learn about Me the More I Understand You

We can use our own experience as the basis for compassion for others. Most therapists don't talk about this with their patients, but the truth is that good therapists have done their own healing work and continue to tend to their own painful experiences as they arise. That very work is the basis for our compassion for others, as well as our ability to see and understand the suffering that our patients experience. We understand their suffering, not just because of theoretical orientations and the substantial conceptual learning we do in our training. The bottom line is that we understand each other's suffering through knowing our own suffering. We may never have had major depression, but we know sadness. We may never have had panic attacks, but we know anxiety and hopelessness. We may never have gone through a divorce, but we've gone through breakups, disagreements, and other losses. We may never have had delusions, but we know what it is like to be confused. And of course, many of us *have* experienced these things ourselves.

When we have the courage to open up to our own painful and scary places, we have the courage to be with others in their painful and scary places. As I often explain to my patients, what we cannot tolerate in ourselves we cannot tolerate in others. If I'm sad and I can't tolerate my own sadness, then I can't be with you when you are sad, because your sadness will remind me of my own and I won't be able to tolerate that. So I'll do whatever I have to do to get you to stop being sad around me. I may try to fix you, shame you, or abandon you— whatever it takes! That's why good therapists have done, and continue to do, the work to heal ourselves. It's why you feel so safe with us. We can go there with you because we can go there with ourselves. And, while it is helpful to have the support of others, the practice of self-compassion really changes everything. With a good, solid self-compassion practice we do have the courage to face whatever we need to face. And that actually connects us to others. We can better understand and hold each other when we know we have self-compassion to hold ourselves.

Of course, this isn't just limited to therapists. This is true for all of us in our daily relationships. Parents can't tolerate in their children what they can't tolerate in themselves, for example. We have a hard time being with friends or loved ones who have feelings we can't tolerate in ourselves. Are you beginning to see how we are interconnected and how facing what is hard for me to face in myself doesn't affect just me? Do you see how having compassion for ourselves is the root of being there for others? The same is true for you in your relationships, whether they be with your partner or a stranger on the street. We can recognize and be with others when they are in pain because we can tolerate our own. When we learn to meet ourselves with self-compassion, we offer ourselves the support we wish to receive from others. And that strengthens our capacity to be compassionate, whether we need to shine that flashlight of compassion outward toward others or inward toward ourselves.

Some people have a hard time with the label *self-compassion*, mostly because it has the word *self* in it. This is especially true in Buddhist circles in which the "self" is often spoken of as something to be transcended. As my friend and colleague Dr. Chris Germer likes to say, "Self-compassion dissolves the self." When, through our own experience of suffering, we come to know the nature of suffering, and through the practice of self-compassion, we come to know the nature of compassion, we begin to understand the universal truth of suffering and compassion. We aren't alone in our suffering or our need for compassion. Compassion for ourselves naturally leads to compassion for others. The truth is self-compassion could just as easily be labeled *inner compassion*. Compassion is just compassion. And we need to be able to shine the light of compassion wherever it is needed. So please don't get hung up on the labels. Every one of us struggles in life, and every one of us needs compassion.

From Me to We

Whether you are on the end of the spectrum that feels isolated or the side that feels responsible for others, the truth is that you matter. I often think of our system of first and last names as a good illustration of this system of belonging. For example, "Michelle Becker" signifies two things. The "Michelle" part honors the part of me that is unique. The part with my own particular way of being in the world—the part of me that, like a snowflake, isn't exactly like any other being on this planet, past, present, or future. That part matters. No one else on this planet could bring exactly what I bring to relationships.

I'm also a Becker. I'm part of a system of interconnections called *family.* The "Becker" part of my name signifies that I'm not alone, that I belong to something larger than myself. It honors the part of me that is bigger than my own needs and desires. It reminds me that I have a responsibility to something beyond myself, that my actions will impact others as their actions impact me. Because we are interconnected, I must consider my impact on others. I cannot be well without the whole Becker system being well.

The point is that they need to be taken together. I need to be both a Michelle and a Becker. If I were just a Michelle and free to do or be whatever I wanted in any moment, I'd be satisfied in one way, but I'd lack a sense of connection and belonging. I'd lack a secure base from which to venture out into the world. Being connected to safe others—colleagues, friends, or family—actually gives me the courage to be more fully myself in the world. When I inevitably fail at something, I have a safe place to land. So being a Becker actually supports my being more fully Michelle.

And if I were just a Becker with a sense of connection and belonging, I'd be happy with the sense of connection and belonging but in some ways might not feel I even existed. Without the Michelle part, it would feel more like I was owned by the Becker part, rather than belonging to it. How could I truly belong if there was no Michelle in the Becker? It is in being my unique self *and* being loved and belonging to a bigger whole that I flourish and the family system flourishes. The Becker system also benefits from my unique way of being in the world. The system is strengthened by my belonging. When we leave others out of our awareness or invite them to belong by becoming the same as us, they can never truly feel like they belong, and we miss out on their unique gifts and talents that could strengthen the system. Diversity and inclusion strengthen the system if we let them.

Beyond even the Becker system, I am part of something much larger, as are you. We are all part of the human family. And the human family is stronger when each individual is stronger. It reminds me of the African concept of *ubuntu.* Ubuntu stems from the understanding that our fate is bound up with the fate of all of humanity. We are part of a whole, and we must keep in mind that our actions impact the health of humanity. I'm told that in some places in Africa if you ask a person how he is, he will respond "We are well" or "We are not so well right now." Maybe his grandmother is ailing. So, in recognition of their interconnectedness, the reply "We are not so well right now" accurately notes the fact that the system is stressed.

At the same time, how could the system be well if *you* are unwell? The system needs your gifts too. In an interview with Tim Modise, Nelson Mandela noted, "Ubuntu does not mean that people should not address themselves. The question therefore is, are you going to do so in order to enable the community around you, and enable it to improve? These are important things in life. And if you can do that, you have done something very important." If you care about others, you cannot leave yourself out of the equation.

I hope you are getting a sense that everyone matters. That's the basis of common humanity. Everyone matters. Everyone belongs. When we really open to the shared human condition, we understand the importance of self-compassion along with compassion. Tending to our own well-being doesn't mean ignoring the needs of others. On the contrary, it means when we ourselves are well we can behave in ways that benefit others. When we practice self-compassion instead of reactivity, our relationships benefit because we can choose to respond in ways that benefit our partners and our relationships. Remember that old saying "If Momma ain't happy, ain't nobody happy"? It has its roots in common humanity, but it's incomplete. The truth is that if everyone in the system isn't happy, the system isn't well. That's why we must work toward a more egalitarian system in our homes, in our countries, and in the world. As long as some are oppressed or left behind, the system isn't well. We need ubuntu. And ubuntu includes you. And me. Every one of us matters. We all have the potential to improve the shared human condition.

If I think about common humanity as along a spectrum of belonging, as shown on page 132, Michelle Becker sits right in the middle of the spectrum. It honors the uniqueness of the individual, and it uses that sense door (my own experiences) to understand and honor others. Both ends of the spectrum—the one that focuses too much on myself and the one that focuses too much on others—leave me isolated. It is only including ourselves in our circle of compassion that gives us a true, balanced sense of belonging. Then we can truly understand common humanity and build our capacity for compassion for whoever needs it.

Belonging

Audio Track 16

Call to mind a friend or someone you admire. Take a moment to focus on what you admire about that person, their particular strengths. Let yourself open to their good qualities.

Like all people, your friend also has struggles and areas where they are trying or need to grow. Take a moment to notice those too. Notice that even though your friend struggles at times, they are in your heart and you are connected.

In your mind's eye, picture them in a place of honor. Maybe you've invited them into your living room, or maybe it is in a meadow or clearing in the forest—whatever feels right to you.

Now call to mind others whom you admire and want to invite into your heart.

One by one, open to their good qualities, and also their struggles and growth edges.

Accept them as they are and then put them in that place of honor along with the first person.

With each person, become aware of how much they matter to you and also how they belong in the world. How their presence matters, even if they are marginalized in some way. See their worthiness.

As you picture this group of people that matter to you, you might imagine them in a circle.

Now imagine them turning toward you.

Imagine that they also see and understand you right now, even the parts you don't show other people or can't see yourself. They see your good qualities—your love of nature or quirky sense of humor, for example.

Take a moment to listen for what they admire about you.

This group also sees your struggles in life and accepts you as you are.

Take a moment to listen as they acknowledge what you struggle with.

And as the group invites you into their circle, they remind you that you matter too. You don't need to wait to be some better version of yourself. You already belong.

You belong because you are fully human, with strengths and struggles. You belong to this group, this circle, and you belong to humanity—just as you are.

Humanity needs what you have to offer, no matter how small you think that is.

Picture yourself joining them in the circle now. You are wanted and welcome. You matter. You belong.

Take a moment now to notice how it feels to recognize that you are not separate. You can be both fully yourself—your unique expression in the world—and also belong.

If you like, take a moment to write about what you experienced and what you would like to remember when you are feeling all alone and have forgotten that you matter, too.

Please don't worry if it was difficult to open fully to the experience of being seen and belonging. It can take some time. I trust that as you continue to practice you too will come to be able to see and accept yourself. No need to rush. Trust yourself.

The invitation to each of us is to take our seat at the table of humanity. When we know that all beings matter—and that includes us—it makes it a bit easier to offer ourselves our own love and affection. And if we have that, we never have to go without love and affection again. We move from the question "Do I matter *to you?*" to the knowledge that by virtue of being born we do matter—as all beings do. And we begin to take our place in our lives and relationships with a sense of dignity and worthiness.

Common Humanity in Three Directions

When you look at how common humanity shows up in your relationship, what do you see? Who belongs? Do people get to be fully themselves and still be loved and belong? Or does the relationship tend to revolve around one of you more than both of you? Healthy relationships are a place where both people feel safe to be fully themselves, where both feel safe being vulnerable, and where everyone feels that they matter and belong. Let's look at that more closely now.

Do You Matter?

While each of us, of course, wants to feel that we matter, that we are accepted and belong just as we are, it doesn't always feel that way. As we saw in Part I of this book, there are so many reasons we get caught in the stress response and in resistance. Your partner gets caught in those things too. As much as she might want to, she can't always be there for you. Like each of us, your partner has needs and desires to tend to.

Another reason we don't always get the care we want from our partners is that in an effort to shield and protect ourselves we don't always allow ourselves to be vulnerable. We don't show that we are hurt or insecure or whatever the vulnerable feeling may be. And if we don't let our partners see us as we are, how can we expect them to know when we need some help or support?

While we are often wishing for care and support from others, we can't *make* others be there for us. We can, however, matter to ourselves. We can commit to always being there for ourselves, ready with understanding, acceptance, compassion, encouragement, just when we need it most.

We also teach people how to treat us, so if we are living life as if we don't matter we will have inadvertently taught those around us that we don't matter. So the real question here isn't whether you matter to your partner. That is important, of course. The more important question, however, is whether you matter to yourself. Can you, will you, show up for yourself? Do you include yourself in your own circle of compassion?

Does Your Partner Matter?

In the section above I noted some of the things that get in the way of your partner's being there for you. Now let's look at what gets in the way of your being there for your partner.

Reactivity

As we've explored in Part I of this book, whenever we feel unsafe, we are wired to react in ways designed to restore safety: fighting, withdrawing, and placating. When we are in this state of reactivity, we treat our partners as if they are the threat. In this state we forget that this person matters to us. That we care about *their* well-being too. In this state we may focus only on ourselves—"I have to get out of here" or "Why can't you see how hurt I am? I deserve to be treated better than this," for example. Or we may focus only on our partner: "You're such a jerk—I can't believe you did that again!" (blaming) or "You're right, you deserve better—would you like a back rub?" (placating). The point is that both people matter. In common humanity we recognize that it isn't me or you. It's both of us.

Resistance

Also in Part I, we looked at how we feel our partners' pain through empathic resonance. And how when we feel overwhelmed by that pain we often move into resistance by fixing, controlling, or criticizing. As human as it is to move into that space of resistance, when we are in that space we are really trying to get out of our own pain by getting our partners out of pain. So even though on the surface it may look like we are focused on our partners—even sacrificing some of our own needs in the process—the truth is usually that it is a strategy to get ourselves out of pain in the end. Our partners don't usually appreciate being fixed, controlled, or criticized. They just want to know we are with them, we love them, and they have our support. And that means opening to and accepting them as they are—in pain and all—rather than trying to relieve our own pain by changing them. They just want to know they matter to us.

Isolation: It's Just Me

We can also get stuck in focusing on our own pain. We see our own end of the equation, how hard it is to miss work again to care for the kids when our partners are sick—especially when there is an important project that needs our attention, for example. We can be so focused on our own discomfort that we forget to notice that our partners are having a hard time too. And when we focus on the burden we are carrying, our partners can feel more of a burden than a blessing. We have forgotten that our partners are people who are also having a difficult time. We have forgotten that their well-being also matters to us. And they will likely get the message that they don't matter to us.

Having practices that help you remember that your partner matters to you, so that you are able to honor and support them as needed, can be really helpful. Mostly what is helpful is anything that helps your partner feel seen, accepted, and loved. Making it a point, for example, to find a regular time to ask them about what happened in their day or to give them a hug or kiss hello/goodbye, or remembering to tell them you love and appreciate them, can go a long way toward letting your partner know they matter to you.

> Even the smallest rituals—a kiss goodbye before you leave for work, a question about how your partner's day went after work—can help your partner feel seen, accepted, and loved.

Does Your Relationship Matter?

Even when we remember that we matter and our partners matter, we can forget that there is a third aspect at play—the relationship. Relationships need care and feeding to survive. When we neglect the relationship, it slowly withers, and years later we can find ourselves wondering what happened to it. As we feel increasingly isolated we wonder, where did it go?

We can find ourselves drawing on the relationship for strength to face the important and urgent circumstances in our life—like caring for an infant, the seemingly constant deadlines at work, the stress of moving or of a parent who requires care, for example. We can take the relationship for granted, not noticing that that relationship also needs care and feeding. We need to share laughter, joy, connection, understanding. Do you know what your relationship needs? Are you finding time to invest in keeping your relationship healthy and satisfying? It can be helpful to have practices that remind you that your relationship matters too. Scheduling regular date nights, for example, can help to regularly invest in the relationship, so that it doesn't just fade away in the stress of managing everyday tasks.

As you reflect upon these three directions of common humanity and belonging, you may have noticed that one or more of them is lacking in your day-to-day life. The following is a practice that, when done regularly, helps to remind us that we matter, our partners matter, and the relationship matters.

TRY THIS

Loving-Kindness for Couples

Audio Track 17

Find a comfortable place to sit or lie down. Take a few moments to settle into feeling supported by your external supports, like the chair, cushion, or floor beneath you.

Then take a few minutes to invite a sense of internal support. You might greet yourself with an inner smile of welcome, place a hand over your heart or elsewhere as a physical gesture of support and kindness, or tune in to your body, breathing with an awareness of how the breath is nourishing you with every inhalation.

If it feels right, call to mind an image or felt sense of yourself as you are right now.

It may help to remember the friends who invited you into their circle in the last exercise. Can you see yourself through their eyes and see how you are worthy of belonging? This group of friends and loved ones sees you as you are and cares about you. They want the best for you. They begin to offer you kind wishes. Perhaps the kind wishes are:

- May you be happy
- May you be peaceful
- May you be healthy
- May you live with ease

Perhaps they are wishes that speak to you more specifi-
cally.

As you feel ready, begin to offer yourself your own kind
wishes:

- May I be happy
- May I be peaceful
- May I be healthy
- May I live with ease

You can use these words or other words that speak more
directly to your situation.

As you say these words silently to yourself, repeating
them over and over, offer them with the intention of kindness
as best you can. No need to rush through them. Say them
slowly and with a warm tone.

When it feels right to move on, call to mind your partner.
You might picture them in your mind or just have a felt sense
of them.

Let yourself feel how much you want them to be happy
and free from suffering.

When you feel ready, offer these phrases (or other ones
if you prefer) to the image of your partner—slowly and gently.

- May you be happy
- May you be peaceful
- May you be healthy
- May you live with ease

As you say these phrases, let yourself feel how much you
care about them and wish them well.

And finally, form a picture or felt sense of you and your
partner together. Allow yourself to know how important your
relationship with this person is.

As you feel ready, begin offering the phrases (or your
own) to both of you:

- May we be happy
- May we be peaceful

- May we be healthy
- May we live with ease

Then let go of the images and phrases and take a moment to notice how you feel right now.

As best you can, accept yourself and your practice just like this, at least for right now.

How did your practice go? If you found that your heart opened a bit and it helped you to remember that you matter, your partner matters, and your relationship matters, see if you can find a way to include the practice in your daily routine. It can be as long or short as you like; the important thing is to do the practice regularly.

If you found the practice difficult or challenging in some way, please be creative in customizing it for yourself. You may want to change the words of the kind wishes, for example. Or you may want to have your eyes closed or open. If it feels too intense to practice in a more meditative way, you could also lighten the practice up by just saying the phrases out loud as you go about the tasks of the day, perhaps when you are stopped at a red light, for example. Be skillful in taking the time to find a way to practice that really works for you.

The point of this practice is not the good feelings that often arise. Those are pleasant and help us know that what we are practicing is what we want to cultivate. The point of the practice is to strengthen the intention of meeting ourselves, our partners, and our relationships with kindness. It reminds us that all three things matter to us. Then, when the stress of life is in full force, we have a better chance of remembering to pause and respond in a way that honors our own needs, our partners' needs, and our relational needs.

It's also a good way to practice cultivating kindness—the subject of the next chapter.

8

Getting What We Need

Kindness in Three Directions

What wisdom can you find that is greater than kindness?
—JEAN-JACQUES ROUSSEAU

I was a couple of days into a mindfulness retreat. It had been a tough beginning for me as I saw the teachers favor one cute, petite, young, and pretty woman in the front row, while being rather harsh with many other participants who had asked questions during the question-and-answer session. On a deeper level it touched a painful scenario from my childhood. I wasn't feeling safe. If those brave enough to ask questions weren't safe, I knew I wouldn't dare speak up during the question-and-answer period.

I was sitting cross-legged in the middle of a big hall with hundreds of people. I'd done my best to be as comfortable as possible—rather, to be less uncomfortable. There was this achy, stabbing, throbbing pain in my hip, and I was tired, cold, and hungry. There were no more pillows to use to prop up my knee, so I found one of the few remaining blankets and folded it up under my knee to relieve the pressure on my sore hip. It helped a bit, but I was still uncomfortable.

It was freezing in the hall, and we were in silence. Well, we were supposed to be in silence. Moments before a woman had come and told me I should give her the blanket I had under my knee because she was cold. I was floored. There were hundreds of people in this hall, many with extra blankets or pillows, and *I* was the one she thought should give up my blanket? She'd come from across the room and made a beeline for me. She didn't care that we were in silence. She didn't care that I was in silence. She just didn't want to be uncomfortable herself. She was cold, she said, and she needed my blanket. And she wasn't going away without my giving it to her. I gave it to her. Sure, there was a small part of me that felt some kindness and generosity—some compassion for her. I truly didn't want her to be cold. But the larger part of me was really resentful. Why were her needs more important than mine? Of course, this touched a much larger theme in my life—everyone else's needs were always more important than mine, or so I had been trained to believe.

Luckily the bell rang to start the meditation. As I opened to what was here for me, I felt the pain in my hip. It wasn't a small pain. But there was a larger pain I felt, the pain of always being overlooked. The pain of always being expected to put my own needs on hold because someone else's needs were more important. I didn't actually buy this idea that others' needs were always more important. Sometimes their needs were more like preferences, when mine were true needs. But the real problem was that I'd been trained not to have needs, not even to see them. And if I did see them, then not to honor them. Effectively, I'd been trained not to matter. And it's one thing not to matter to others, but not to matter to oneself? That's a tragedy.

The Arising of Kindness

As I opened to the pain of never mattering, a fierceness of love and caring arose within me. I *refused* to be overlooked. I saw the amount of suffering that came from being overlooked, and my heart opened for all people everywhere who are overlooked—and also for myself. I couldn't do anything about whether others saw me or turned away, but I could do something about how I showed up. No matter who else turned away, *I would not turn away ever again*. I would see myself, my joys and my sorrows, all of it. I knew in the deepest way possible that it wasn't just others who mattered—*I mattered too*. And a tenderness arose. A *caring* arose. I began to incline gently toward myself. As I went through the days and weeks that followed I found myself asking,

"What do *you* want for lunch, Michelle?" "Where would *you* like to go?" "What shall we do next?" Wherever I went, there was a kind and compassionate presence that went with me. A part that saw, cared about, and tended to myself.

The Arrival of Self-Compassion

And that really changed everything. Eventually, it even changed my relationships. In the beginning I experienced more of the softer side of self-compassion, the nurturing side. I found that I could open to the pain I was experiencing—especially because when I did, *there was someone there who cared.* It was now actually safe to open to my own feelings. I didn't depend on others being there for me—something that had previously been unpredictable. And something else happened too. It gave me the courage to speak up for myself. Beyond that softer and more nurturing side, there was a fierce and protective side. A side that did not want to participate in harm—harm to myself or anyone else. I'd found a strong back. I'd long had a side that wasn't what I would call outright rebellious. It was more a "spunky" side. It was a side that was willing to push back at times. But that side was more rooted in reactivity than in responsiveness. *This* strong back was truly rooted in care and could see the truth of the situation, the bigger picture.

The Relational Effects of Self-Compassion

When I became unwilling to tolerate harm, my relationships changed. This new way of being was far from the "be nice" strategy I was taught as a young girl that was ostensibly a strategy to belong, but that really left me disenfranchised, disconnected, and powerless. Instead, this new way of being left me empowered, authentic, and kind. It gave me the resilience to be able to open to caring about other people too, like that person who demanded my blanket. As I became both fierce and tender in self-compassion I found myself moving from a feeling of irritation toward her to a feeling of tenderness and care toward her. Compassion was no longer a scarce commodity. The more compassion

I gave myself, the more compassion I had for others. Most people don't really see the fierce side of compassion and how it supports our capacity to be tender toward others. Rather, people tend to see things as kindness versus harshness.

Understanding Self-Kindness

Kristin Neff talks about self-kindness as the third component of self-compassion. She goes on to describe self-kindness as the opposite of self-judgment and to talk about what we do when things go wrong in our lives. How do we respond to ourselves? Do we find an inner ally that is kind and supportive? Do we meet ourselves with a kind and supportive touch and some understanding, as in the Putting Self-Compassion into Practice exercises in Chapter 5? Or do we hear a judgmental and harsh voice—one that blames us, calls us names, and tells us to stop being such a wuss and just get on with things? This is really the self-kindness versus self-judgment dilemma.

Just like the other two components, mindfulness and common humanity, I see self-kindness along a spectrum, as depicted below. On one end of the spectrum there is plenty of warmth and softness, but we can tend toward self-indulgence, which isn't actually kind. On the other end there is the fierceness of self-judgment. Self-indulgence feels good, at least in the moment, but it isn't actually good for us. Self-kindness sits in the middle of the spectrum and tends to our well-being, or eudemonia. What is truly kind isn't just what feels good in this moment. It requires a longer-term view of things, to consider what will actually be good for us, what is actually kind.

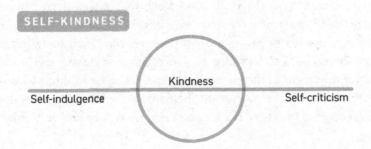

Most of us have a tendency toward self-indulgence or self-judgment, often depending on what we experienced in our family of origin. If our parents tended to indulge us, out of a misguided notion of love or out of a strategy to appease us so that they didn't have to deal with our needs, we will likely tend toward self-indulgence—confusing it with true kindness. Or, if our parents were on the neglectful side, because they didn't have the skills to parent well or because they were working hard to provide for us, we may also associate self-indulgence with self-kindness. True self-kindness, however, gives us what we need, rather than what we want when we want it.

If we had a parent who was critical of us, either because they were just discharging their pain onto us or because they were trying to make us the best we could be in a misguided effort to offer us love, it is likely that we will have a self-critical voice that picks up criticizing us where they left off. This too can be confusing. We may wonder whether the criticism is our only way to motivate ourselves to achieve our goals. True self-kindness does notice when we are not doing well, but it motivates us to achieve our goals with encouragement and love rather than harsh self-criticism.

Of course, as Neff suggests, self-judgment and the resulting self-criticism are the most common opposites of self-kindness. It's what happens when our fierceness toward ourselves is rooted in fear rather than love. It's also what happens when our drive system is activated and isn't rooted in the care system. If we try to avoid pain by working hard, we may find ourselves driven by a harsh inner critic, as Mel did.

From Critical to Caring: The Story of Mel

Mel was sixty-something before learning what self-kindness really is. Having grown up in the Hollywood scene with a somewhat famous parent, Mel was really sensitive to the need to belong—and the price one needed to pay to belong. Between the "ideal body" ideas of Hollywood—and, let's face it, just about everywhere else—and Mel's involvement in the medical field and desire for health, Mel was determined not to be overweight. Being overweight might mean not being accepted by others, but it also might mean poor health. Neither outcome was acceptable. So, Mel meticulously tended to diet and exercise. Friends often remarked that they couldn't believe how Mel could stick to such an austere diet.

Growing up in the celebrity world can have a dark side. Mel's parents were often critical of the way Mel looked or behaved—and when they were drinking, the criticism was quite caustic. "People will never like you," "You're worthless," "You're lazy," and "Fix your hair!" were the kinds of things they'd spew at Mel. They thought that would provide motivation. And it did, but it was motivation based in fear. As Mel grew up, self-criticism took center stage as a way to achieve things. Mel heard, "You're fat," "Don't be such a loser," "You have no willpower," and "People will never like you" after eating something not on the diet. Only this time, the voice was coming from the inside. That didn't make it any less painful. It was a near-constant barrage, and it undermined Mel's sense of well-being and confidence. More than that, Mel became obsessed with diet and exercise, miserable, and unhealthy.

Our work together helped Mel see where this inner critic came from—and the effects it had on Mel's well-being. And we began to explore a different way of being—one that trusted Mel's essential goodness, forgave the mistakes, and was rooted in truly caring about well-being. Gradually, Mel began to tend to diet and exercise from a place of love. "Because I love you and I don't want you to suffer" became the voice that motivated Mel to avoid that sugary piece of chocolate cake rather than the voice that said, "Don't be such a loser." Over time Mel became happier and healthier. Sure, there was an initial phase where Mel went a little too far into self-indulgence. But over time Mel landed squarely in the middle of the spectrum—in self-kindness and eudemonic well-being rather than the hedonism of self-indulgence or the self-flagellation of self-criticism. And something else happened too. Mel's relationships shifted. Mel had always been put off by the sugary-sweet niceness of other people—it felt too much like self-indulgence and was not to be trusted. Now Mel began to see that those relationships that were based in harshness and criticism toward Mel were not appealing either. Mel wanted authenticity—the truth—but not the brutal truth. Truth that came out of a place of kindness. Relationships that were rooted in respect and authenticity.

Finding the Self-Compassionate Voice

As we look at self-kindness and self-compassion, it's worth taking some time to notice how we relate to ourselves. If you too find there is a harsh inner critic always ready to judge you, or if you find an inner voice that charms you into self-indulgence, you may find the following exercise helpful. As always, please engage at whatever level feels right for you. This exercise is an adaptation of the Finding Your Compassionate Voice exercise in the MSC program and can sometimes move us outside our window of tolerance (see Chapter 6), so please feel free to skip it or otherwise disengage if that feels right. You can always come back to it when you feel ready.

TRY THIS
Motivating Yourself with Compassion

Audio Track 18

Consider a behavior you often engage in that really isn't serving you and in fact often gets in the way of your well-being. Something you would like to change.

Perhaps you overeat at times or procrastinate. Or maybe you don't exercise or meditate as often as you would like. Maybe you're too reactive, often getting angry at people who are just trying to help you. Or perhaps you've been too flirty with others even though you are in a monogamous, committed relationship.

As with all our practices, see if you can stay in the mild to moderate range in choosing something to work with here. Choose something important enough that you can feel it, but not something that is overwhelming for you.

We learn best by building strength while staying within our window of tolerance.

When you have that behavior in mind, please write it down.

Please consider why you would like to change the behavior:

- What is continuing to behave this way costing you?
- How do you imagine life would be better without this behavior?
- Why do you want to change?

Now notice how you feel when you indulge in that behavior:

- What happens *just before* you indulge? If you didn't indulge, what would you be feeling? Is indulging in this behavior a way of changing your feelings?
- What happens *while* you are indulging? What does it feel like? Are these your desired feelings? Is there any cost while you are indulging?
- What happens *after* you indulge? Is there a price that you pay? Is there harm to yourself? Your partner? Your relationship?

Please write down what you find.

Become aware of how you relate to yourself when you behave this way.

Is there an inner voice that charms and indulges you?

- What does this voice say to you? "Go ahead; you deserve it," "It won't matter," "I'll start tomorrow," or something else?
- If you have an inner voice that encourages self-indulgence, please write down what it says.
- Now consider whether this voice is actually helping you achieve your goals. Is it helping or causing you harm?
- Even though this voice often leads you astray, please consider whether there is a kind intention underneath this voice. Is it trying to offer you ease, comfort, pleasure?
- Please write down any kind intention you find.

Is there an inner voice that judges, shames, or criticizes you?

- What does this voice say to you? "You can't do anything right," "You're a loser," "You're worthless," or something else?
- If you have an inner critical voice, please write down what it says.
- Now consider whether this voice is actually helping you achieve your goals. Is it helping or causing you harm?
- Even though this voice may be causing you harm, please consider whether there is a kind intention underneath this voice. Is it trying to help you in some way? Does it want you to be safe, healthy, lovable?
- Please write down any kind intention you find.

Note: Sometimes this harsh voice isn't actually trying to help you; it is just a repetition of a harmful voice from someone in your life. In this case, it may be best to skip giving voice to this part and go directly to finding your compassionate voice.

As you become aware of the inner indulgent or critical voice (or both!) and the kind intentions underneath, please take a moment to acknowledge the efforts of this part of yourself that has worked very hard to try to help you, even though the result has been harmful.

- If it feels right, freely and spontaneously write a letter to that part of yourself, acknowledging its efforts to be helpful and letting it know it doesn't have to continue in that role. We'll soon be finding a compassionate voice to support achieving our goals.

Now that the inner indulgent and critical voices have been acknowledged, invite them to take a step back and allow space for the inner compassionate voice to arise. This part sees you, understands you, and wants the best for you. It is concerned with your well-being and happiness, and it is willing to do what is needed to ensure your success in the long run. It can see how the behavior is causing you harm, and it wants you to stop. It doesn't think something is wrong with you; rather, it understands why you sometimes get caught in the behavior, and it still wants you to stop, *because you are worthy of being well, healthy, happy, loved—whatever you find you truly need.* This inner compassionate voice comes from a place of love.

- Please take a few minutes and write a letter to yourself from the inner compassionate voice.
- Let the compassionate voice speak to the behavior you want to change, why it is important, and the steps you'd like to take.
- Most of all, let the inner compassionate voice speak to you from a place of love.

How did it feel to motivate yourself from a place of kindness and compassion, rather than self-indulgence or self-judgment? You might keep the letter handy and read it daily to support keeping yourself on the path to changing your behavior. We want to reinforce the capacity to relate to ourselves with true kindness rather than self-indulgence or self-judgment.

Self-Compassion: Soft and Strong

We might think of these ends of the self-kindness spectrum—self-indulgence and self-judgment—as the soft front and strong back from Chapter 4. Self-indulgence often arises when we allow our feelings—especially the desire for pleasure—to run the show. On the other hand, when we approach ourselves with only strength and determination, we may find our approach to be too harsh and critical.

Soft Front

On one end of the spectrum, the soft front holds the capacity for comforting, soothing, and validating us. Comforting is often physical compassion, soothing is emotional compassion, and validating is mental compassion. This soft place to land, so to speak, allows us to be vulnerable. And vulnerability is important—it is what is required for us to be known, seen, understood, and loved. If we don't know who we really are and what we really feel, how on earth could we know how to tend to ourselves? And if we don't show others who we really are and what we really feel, how could they know what we truly need?

Strong Back

On the other end of the spectrum, the strong back holds the functions of providing, protecting, and motivating ourselves. Is it any less kind to tend to our needs by going out in the world and working for what we need—food, clothing, shelter, and so on? Or by protecting ourselves, both physically, by taking cover or fighting when we are under attack, and emotionally, by setting limits and saying no, even leaving harmful relationships? And is finding the motivation and the encouragement to follow our dreams and tend to our needs by sticking with things that are hard any less compassionate? We need this strong back just as much as the soft front. But that isn't usually what we think of when we think of self-kindness. So often we think of compassion as something rather soft and fluffy. And that may be something you long for, or something that turns your stomach like it used to for Mel. Both are common reactions.

The Full Spectrum of Self-Kindness

Depending on the experiences in our lives, we may be lacking more of the softness or more of the strength of compassion. There is a danger in being too soft, as there is in being too strong. Actually, it's not that it is too soft or too strong per se, more that it is *only soft or strong*. True self-compassion has the capacity for both and is rooted in the wisdom of mindfulness. True self-compassion sees what is needed here—what is truly kind, not just what feels good—and can respond with both strength and softness. It's what Germer and Neff refer to as the "caring force" in the MSC program.

It's likely that our strong back or soft front tendencies also are influenced by the things we learned from our parents. We may have developed really helpful qualities, and we may also be lacking the capacity to be vulnerable (soft front) or to have the confidence to stand up for what we need and set limits with others (strong back).

When we land on the end of the spectrum with too much soft-ness and not enough strength, we can easily become flooded by our emotions. We ruminate, and we often go into overwhelm. We get caught in our own problems, and we become disconnected from oth-ers or caught in others' problems and disconnected from ourselves. We find ourselves here when we've been trained to be "nice" rather than to be kind by also tending to our own well-being. Without the clear seeing of mindfulness and the strength of the strong back, we become impulsive. And without the strong back, we collapse. Self-indulgence lives in this place of softness without strength.

However, when we have the vulnerability of the soft front sup-ported by the strength of the strong back, we can feel things, and that helps us recognize and accept the reality of things. We can cultivate a steadiness or equanimity with our openness. It allows for healing and resilience and for us to be nourished. And it forms the basis for healthy connection with others—and with ourselves. We need the support of the strong back to safely open to the soft front—our vulnerability and the basis for our connection.

And just as the soft front needs the strong back, the strong back also needs the vulnerability of the soft front. When we are all strength and no vulnerability, we become rigid, inflexible, and brittle. We lack the feeling that informs good decision making and underlies our capac-ity to be with things and to heal from our previous wounds. We end up stuffing down our feelings and dragging around a suitcase of old hurts. And it takes quite a lot of energy to drag around that invisible suitcase of hurt! When we push away the vulnerability of the soft front, we push away our feelings—all feelings, even joy. We inadvertently push away the possibility of healing those hurts and emptying the suitcase. We also need to push away others who remind us of our hurts—lest the feelings arise in us again. We find ourselves strong—and isolated. Self-judgment lives in this place of fierceness without softness.

However, when that strength is combined with the vulnerability of the soft front, we have the strength we need to open to the truth of things and the resilience we need to face them and heal from them. This is what I found when I was on retreat. Far from the habit of stoicism that I was raised with (as are most Scandinavians), I had to open to the pain I was in before I could begin to heal it. When our strength is combined with the vulnerability of the soft front, there is groundedness, stability, and the capacity to endure. Like the willow tree whose branches can bend with the wind, we are much more likely to endure the storms of our lives when we're able to bend and flex than if we were only strong, hard, and rigid, without the capacity to bend and flex. There is courage to open to what we need to face rather than pushing things away in order to feel strong. Experts call this *psychological flexibility*, and studies have found that it is at the heart of healthy relationships.

When we can tend to ourselves with kindness, we can help ourselves move from the reactivity of the fight/flight/freeze system to the care system with its sense of safeness and affiliation. From this place it is much easier to determine our best course of action. And it is much easier to be able to take in what our partners are saying and what they need. In other words, when we take the time to notice and tend kindly to our own suffering, we create the opportunity to tend to our partners and our relationships from a much wiser place. The following practice, adapted from the MSC program, may be helpful.

> Tending to ourselves with kindness helps us move from the threat/defense system to the care system and respond to our partners from a much wiser place.

TRY THIS
Soften, Soothe, and Allow

Audio Track 19

Call to mind a situation that is causing you some distress. This could be a relational problem, especially with your partner, or it could be any situation. All kinds of problems are okay here because all kinds of practice are helpful. Again, stick to something you can feel in your body, but not something that is overwhelming. Perhaps a 3–4 on a distress scale of 1–10 where 10 is the most stressful.

As you open to the situation, notice how you feel physically, mentally, and emotionally.

- No need to change things or make them go away; just meet yourself with curiosity.
- What is happening in your body? What thoughts are you having? What emotions are present?

Now, opening to the body sensations, see where you feel the distress most easily in your body. Perhaps an achiness in the chest, a tightness in the throat, or a tightening in the belly. See where it is for you.

- If you can, meet that place with some physical compassion.
- Perhaps offer a kind touch by placing your hand on that part of the body. Let the hand fill with kindness and let kindness seep from the hand into the body.
- If you find that the body is holding the tension in an effort to be strong, without much softness, balance that strength with a sense of softness now. Invite a sense of softness and ease into that part of the body.
- No need to force this softening; just allow the body to soften. Perhaps soften around the area of tension or other physical sensation.
- You might even find it helpful to gently whisper to yourself, "Softening, softening, softening."
- Stay here as long as you like.

Now offer some mental compassion. If you find you've been resisting the situation, perhaps with thoughts of "It's not right" or "It shouldn't be like this," see if you can drop the fight with things as they are, offering yourself some ease by allowing things to be as they are.

- Remember, we aren't saying we are okay with the situation or we don't need to do things differently in the future. We are simply acknowledging that in this moment this is how things are and allowing our minds to rest a bit.

- If it feels right, perhaps gently whisper to yourself, "Allowing, allowing, allowing" as you open to the reality of the situation.
- Stay here as long as you like.

And finally, offer some emotional compassion.

- Given whatever emotions are present for you, what do you need to hear? Words of comfort, validation, and reassurance? "You did the best you could," or "I'm here for you," or "Of course you're upset after what you've been through"?
- Or maybe you need to be reminded of your strong back? Perhaps the words you need to hear are more like "You're okay," "You can do this," or "You'll get there."
- Please take some time to offer yourself what you need to hear right now.
- If you are having trouble finding kind words, you might consider what you would say to a dear friend in the same situation. Can you offer yourself a similar message?
- Or perhaps there is someone in your life who always offers you kindness. What would they say to you? Can you let their words in or say them to yourself? If not, just having the intention to be kind and understanding is enough.
- If you did find words, see if you can soften and allow the kind words in.
- If it feels right, perhaps say to yourself, "Soothing, soothing, soothing" as you meet yourself with kindness.
- Stay here as long as you like.

Now take a moment and notice how you feel after tending to yourself this way.

- Was there a part of the practice that was most helpful to you? Physical compassion, mental compassion, or emotional compassion?
- Were there any parts that were harder for you?

- Each practice and each person is different. There is no right or wrong, just whatever is helpful.

- What did you notice about the strong back and the soft front? Did you notice you needed more of the soft front—comfort, validation, and soothing? Or more of the strong back—protections, providing, and motivating? The goal is to have access to both your strength and your vulnerability.

Now you know more about what you need and what you can offer yourself when you find yourself in the midst of difficult emotions.

Please take some time to write down what you learned in this exercise.

Self-kindness really rests on the question "What do I need right now?" It isn't a question of what feels good in the moment, and it isn't a question of bearing anything in the name of achieving our goals. Self-compassion is rooted in mindfulness. We root in and accept things as they are. We understand we are not alone in the struggles of life. Through shared common humanity we know it is normal to struggle, and that it's okay to tend to our own suffering—just not to get caught in the delusion that we are the only ones who have problems. And then, given that we can see our suffering more clearly, we intentionally invite wisdom in by asking what we need right now. What is actually skillful and wise? And as best we can we give ourselves what we truly need, just as we would do for someone else we loved. Like a good mom, we give ourselves what is most likely to lead to true and lasting well-being. And that is truly the kindest path.

> Asking ourselves what we need right now does not mean indulging in momentary desires but, like a good mom, giving ourselves what will lead to lasting well-being.

Kindness in Three Directions

Self-kindness is an essential component of self-compassion. Together with mindfulness and common humanity, it forms a solid foundation of well-being that allows us to engage in the often more challenging task of offering kindness to our partners and our relationships. Let's take a look at how kindness flows in our relationships.

Self-Kindness

Now that we have a better understanding of where we miss true self-kindness and what we need to cultivate, we are much better able to begin meeting ourselves with the kindness we have always needed and deserved. We ask ourselves, "What do I need?" and then we show up for ourselves in ways that are truly kind.

This allows us to engage in our relationships from a place of empowerment rather than dependency. No other person, no matter how much they love us—and even if they want to—can meet all of our needs. Without a solid self-compassion practice we will find ourselves dependent on others for kindness and understanding. And we will feel resentful when they, for whatever reason, aren't able to provide the kindness and compassion we need. With a reliable self-compassion practice, we can meet our own needs, even when others let us down.

The following exercise, adapted from the MSC program, can help you give yourself compassion even when your partner has let you down.

TRY THIS
Meeting Our Own Needs

Audio Track 20

Call to mind a time when you needed something from your partner but didn't get it. A time that left you feeling angry or hurt in some way. Please choose something that was difficult enough that you could feel the emotions, but not something that was traumatic. Stay within your window of tolerance as best you can.

Allow yourself to remember the situation in detail. Who was there or wasn't there? What was said or wasn't said? What happened or didn't happen?

As you remember the situation, see if you can identify the feelings that arose for you.

Some feelings, such as anger, form a protective layer. If anger is present, you might validate your anger, perhaps saying to yourself, "Of course you're angry; anyone would feel angry in that situation." Or whatever feels right to you. The point is not to reinforce the storyline; it is to acknowledge and accept the feelings you are having.

Underneath that protective layer, there is often a softer, more vulnerable layer. Here you may feel something like sadness, embarrassment or shame, disappointment, loneliness. As you identify these softer, more vulnerable feelings, see if you can find the strongest feeling.

Naming the feeling can be very helpful, perhaps saying to yourself with kindness and understanding something like "Loneliness—of course you are feeling lonely" or "Rejection—yes, it does feel like rejection." Underneath the vulnerable feeling there is often an unmet need. This would be a universal human need that by virtue of being human everybody needs. Maybe that is the need to be loved, to be seen, or connected, or to be accepted, for example. See if you can identify what the need is for you.

As best you can, try offering yourself what you need, perhaps saying to yourself, "I see you" if you need to be seen, for example. Or if you need to belong, you might say, "I care about you; you matter to me" or, if you need to feel loved or accepted, perhaps something like "I love you just as you are." See what it is for you. Continue offering yourself your own kindness as long as you need.

What was it like to give yourself what you need? We have the capacity to take care of ourselves even when others aren't available or don't know what we need. When we can count on ourselves for kindness, we are safer in relationship. We can take the risk to be vulnerable because if things don't turn out the way we want we can count on ourselves for comfort and soothing.

When rooted in mindfulness and common humanity, self-kindness turns into self-compassion. When we see ourselves as we are, take our place as part of humanity, and meet ourselves with true kindness and compassion, we have uncovered the inner compassionate voice. Whenever this part of us is active, we have activated the affiliative nature of the care system and are able to tend to our own safeness and well-being—whether through softness or strength or both. We can tolerate the vulnerability required to create true intimacy in relationships, and we can set the limits and boundaries we need when things go awry in the relationship. When we cultivate our own capacity for self-kindness, we need never go without again.

> Cultivating self-kindness means we never have to go without kindness again.

Kindness toward Our Partners: Benefits and Blocks

In previous chapters we've explored being better able to see our partners—especially when they are having a difficult time. We also need to keep in mind that they matter to us—we want them to be happy and free from suffering as much as possible. And there is also another step—the intentional cultivation of kindness toward them. When we see their suffering and remember their importance to us, we need to keep our hearts open to them. With a sense of curiosity we begin to explore the question "What do *you* need?"

Becoming Mindful of Resistance

We need to watch that this question isn't a form of resistance. We don't want to use this question to avoid our partner's pain, as we do when we engage the drive system, especially fixing. We must root in true mindfulness, truly opening to them and turning toward their pain with acceptance. This activates the affiliative system; they are not in it alone. They get a sense of mattering to us. In and of itself, this is an act of kindness when we bear witness to another. Rather than feeling defective and abandoned when we try to fix them, when we have room for them and for their pain they feel loved and valued. We know we are in this place when our hearts are open rather than resistant or closed.

How Common Humanity Connects

Common humanity also softens the heart if we let it. When we hold our partner's humanness alongside our own, there is a sense of connection and concern. We know what it is like to be scared, angry, hurt, reactive. We are familiar with acting unskillfully out of the threat/defense system, rather than out of the safety and contentedness of the care system. And when we've opened to our partner's pain and remembered that they matter to us, a desire to offer compassion arises.

When we land in this open-hearted place, we naturally wonder what they need. Perhaps it is soft and nurturing, like comforting, soothing, or validation. Perhaps it is a strong-back type of need, like motivating them ("You can do it—I believe in you!"), protecting them (standing up to people who are insulting them, for example), or providing for them (taking on more responsibility so that they can have a needed rest).

Finding What Is Truly Kind

An important aspect of kindness toward your partner is to know the difference between what you would want in the situation and what your partner would want. For example, in many relationships one partner feels comforted and soothed by words. Having a conversation and knowing that the other person understands and is supportive comes before wanting the comfort of physical touch, if it is wanted at all. The other person may find words and conversation more challenging and would prefer physical touch. There is no right and wrong here. What is skillful is to know and understand the difference so that you can offer what your partner needs rather than your own preference.

Finding What Is Truly Kind

Bring to mind a time when you were having a difficulty and you turned to your partner and felt very comforted and supported. What did your partner do or say?

Or bring to mind a difficulty you are currently in the midst of and imagine yourself turning toward your partner and receiving the comfort and support you desire. What does your partner do or say?

These are the ways in which your partner can best comfort and soothe you or encourage you. There may be softer aspects like validating, comforting, and soothing or stronger aspects like protecting, providing, or motivating. Take a moment to notice what works best for you. You may want to write about this.

Now bring to mind a scenario in which your partner was having a difficult time. Maybe they turned toward you for support, or maybe they were trying to handle it themselves, but you noticed anyway.

- What types of things did they find comforting and supportive? It's also helpful to notice things they don't find helpful.

- If you don't have a sense of what they find helpful, try experimenting a bit:

  —What if you just stood close to them so they could feel your presence?

  —What if you reached out and offered a hug?

  —What if you acknowledged the situation briefly, perhaps just naming their situation and adding "That's gotta be rough."

  —What if you asked them about it and then listened attentively, without judgment or advice, as they detailed how hard it is for them?

  —What if you offered to take on more of the household tasks so they could have a break?

- These aren't magical solutions, just ideas about how to begin to explore what your partner finds helpful.

- As you continue to explore or remember what they find helpful, notice whether they prefer the softer side (comfort, validation, soothing) or the stronger side (protection, motivation, providing).

Notice the similarities and differences in your styles. You may want to write down what you found.

The next time your partner is having a difficult time, take a moment to remember what they find helpful.

Fine-tuning the capacity to meet one's partner with kindness can turn a downward spiral into an upward spiral. While a moment o kindness can change the course of your evening, a string of such moments can change the quality of your relationship.

> A moment of kindness can change an evening. A string of such moments can change a relationship.

In the Compassion for Couples program we invite couples to have a conversation about what comforts and soothes them with their partner. Many couples find this eye opening and empowering. If your partner is willing, you may also want to have this conversation. If not, just knowing what you and your partner find compassionate can change the situation and the relationship over time.

Kindness in the Relationship

More kindness in the relationship lands the relationship in the care system. Both partners feel safe, content, and connected most of the time. But there is a third entity in relationships: we must look out for the relationship itself. Just like you and your partner, relationships require regular care and feeding and can become distressed.

It's worth taking a moment to notice the state of your relationship.

Has it become routine and dull—lacking a spark? Is it in a state of disrepair and distress? Or is it alive and fulfilling for both partners? Just as we ask, "What do I need?" for ourselves or "What do you need?" for our partners, we can also consider, "What does our relationship need?"

And we can notice the conditions that create well-being in the relationship. If it has become routine and dull, for example, it may be that the relationship needs more attention and adventure or excitement. Perhaps add in shared experiences of going on dates or family adventures. Breaking the routine in ways that allow for both connection and excitement can be really helpful.

Or if the relationship has become distressed, often adding in safety is helpful. Theorists talk about safety as a precondition for compassion. What would it take to restore safety in the relationship? Do some limits or boundaries need to be put in place? Would it be helpful if both partners could count on being seen and valued? Are there gestures of kindness that could help heal some of the wounds? Often working with a skilled couples therapist can provide the needed safety while partners learn how to build a more satisfying relationship.

Or perhaps your relationship is in a really good place right now. If so, that's wonderful! Keeping it that way requires care and attention. What are the things you most value in the relationship? How can you safeguard those things? For example, if you feel loved and connected, perhaps having a regular practice of making space to see and tend to each other would be helpful. Like making it a point to check in with each other over dinner or making sure to talk about your hopes and dreams with each other.

The point of kindness in the relationship is to consider "What does our relationship need?" And then, as best you can, to invest the needed resources in your relationship.

I don't want to give you the idea that kindness is all about the softer side. Even in our relationships the strong side is important. Boundaries, for example, are important—boundaries within the relationship, so that everyone feels safe and gets what they need, and also boundaries between the relationship and the rest of the world so that the relationship is protected from outside interference. We need to protect our relationships. We need to provide for our relationships, by investing time, attention, and other resources in them. And we need to stay motivated to tend to the relationship. When we need to set limits to avoid being harmed, it can feel uncomfortable for both people. Even then, though, it is the kindest thing to do. We don't want to participate in harm.

Putting It All Together

For compassion to blossom, we need mindfulness, common humanity, and kindness, as depicted in the diagram below. We have presented them sequentially here, and they often arise that way. However, for it to truly be compassion all elements need to be present simultaneously. We need to open to things as they are (see clearly), remember everyone matters, and tend to ourselves and each other with kindness.

When all three components are present, compassion is present. And our relationships are characterized by loving (kindness), connected (common humanity) presence (mindfulness).

Cultivating our own capacity to meet ourselves with compassion both empowers us to show up with vulnerability and develop intimacy in our relationships (because we can care for ourselves if we are disappointed) and provides the base of personal experience that helps us better understand our partners. Just as all three elements (mindfulness, common humanity, and kindness) need to be present for

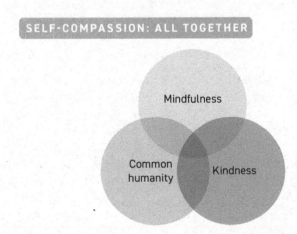

SELF-COMPASSION: ALL TOGETHER

Mindfulness

Common humanity

Kindness

compassion, compassion in our relationships requires tending to all three directions: compassion for ourselves, compassion for our partners, and compassion for our relationships.

Part II has helped us develop a base to do just that. In Part III we turn our attention to putting these practices into action in our relationships.

Part III

Putting It into Practice

Tailoring Compassion Skills
to Your Relationship

In Part I of this book we explored three emotion regulation systems—threat/defense, drive, and care—and how they enter into our relationships. In Part II we looked at how to develop the care system through the three components of self-compassion: mindfulness, common humanity, and kindness. Here in Part III, we will look at how to put those three components into action in our primary relationships. In the next chapter, we take a look at how to root our actions in what is meaningful to us, our partners, and our relationships.

9

"What Really Matters to Us?"

Rooting Your Relationship in Your Values

> If you want to identify me, ask me not where I live, or what
> I like to eat, or how I comb my hair, but ask me what I am
> living for, in detail, and ask me what I think is keeping me
> from living fully for the things I want to live for.
> —THOMAS MERTON

There is that line about marriage: *And the two shall become one.* For many single people this sounds like the answer to their dreams. No longer lonely, no longer incomplete, no longer unsure of their desirability, they will live happily ever after. Each will gain what the other has to offer. No one thinks about what they'll give up in this scenario—until they start the happily ever after part. Then the battle for survival begins. After all, if two people are going to somehow end up becoming one person, someone is going to have to give something up. That's just math!

Most of us don't really draw a distinction between ourselves and our partners. In the effort to achieve the harmony of oneness, we either meld ourselves to what our partners value or see our partners through our own lens. And in a larger sense we sometimes miss what is deeply meaningful to them. We don't see them as separate individuals with their own needs and desires. Then we wonder why they hesitate to enter fully into the relationship.

Other times we are acutely aware that we and our partners are different. And that awareness leads to a battlefield of sorts, where we

173

engage in a tug-of-war, with each of us desperately fighting to pull the other onto our side of what matters. I'm sure it comes as no surprise that all of these strategies at best limit the joy in relationships and at worst create harm for ourselves, our partners, and our relationships.

How the Two Become Three: Discovering You, Me, and Us

It turns out that in healthy relationships two really becomes three: me, you, and us. One sign of a healthy relationship is that both people become *more themselves*. Far from leading them to give up who they are and become less in order to belong, the relationship provides a safety net that allows both partners to risk becoming more fully themselves by going for what is truly meaningful for them.

A real relationship needs to have two whole people in it. That means, in addition to becoming more fully ourselves, we need to see and understand our partners and what they value. It is important that we do our best to help them discover and realize what is deeply important to them. Partners who are deeply satisfied can bring the best of themselves to their relationships.

And how does the relationship become a source of support for each partner? When the partners take the time to discover and honor what the relationship itself needs. When we tend to all three aspects in the relationship, not just in a surface way, but really, truly tend to what is deeply meaningful, we end up with a deeply satisfying relationship, a deeply satisfied partner, *and* a deeply satisfying life. This is the power of wisdom combined with care.

So how do we get to this deeply satisfying life? It begins with opening to ourselves with curiosity. As I read the quote at the top of the chapter I can't help being curious. I wonder what is keeping you from living fully for the things *you* want to live for. Of course to answer that question you'd need to know what it is you are living for. I find this is a topic of some confusion for many of us. It's hard to tend to what matters without actually knowing what that is. It may be helpful to start with an exploration about what values are and are not.

Needs versus Values

As humans we have in common certain needs. We have physical needs like food, clothing, and shelter. And we have emotional needs like the need to be seen, loved, valued, to belong. So it is with our relationships; healthy relationships need trust, honesty, forgiveness, care, and many other things. We've already explored many aspects of building a healthy foundation based on our needs. But relationships, like life, aren't a one-size-fits-all endeavor. Beyond our commonalities that bind us together as humans, we are individuals—each unique. And when two unique people come together and form a relationship, that is unique too. To understand what makes *your* life and *your* relationship worth living for you need to understand what you value.

Values are what give our life meaning. They are what personally matter to us, and they reflect what we want our life to stand for. For example, one might value maintaining a healthy lifestyle, engaging in challenging and fulfilling work, creative expression, living with a sense of adventure, financial stability, or feeling close and connected to others. Accordingly, what brings us happiness, or unhappiness, is often rooted in our core values. Imagine you'd been working at a steady, reliable job making a good income, but the job was rather boring for you. Now imagine you find out that you've been part of a reduction in force and you will be given six weeks of pay but your job is now over. Is this good or bad news? The answer depends on what you value. If you value creative expression, challenging work, or adventure, this may actually feel like a blessing—you've been released from something that was in the way of what you value and are free to pursue what you do value. However, if you value financial stability, this likely is terrible news.

It isn't what happens to us as much as how that impacts what we value that causes us difficulty. Of course, this is true with our needs too. We need safety, for example, so being mugged would be bad news for all of us. The difference is that when we get beyond our universal human needs, what brings us satisfaction or dissatisfaction depends on our personal values.

> What happens to us doesn't cause us as much difficulty as the impact of these experiences on what we value.

Values versus Goals

Another area of confusion around values is what is a value and what is a goal. They are related, but different. Values guide our choices, but we don't choose them; rather we uncover them. We do, however, choose our goals. For example, you might discover that you feel rather alive and happy when you are traveling, exploring new places, and taking on new roles. It's possible that a personal value for you would be something like adventure. Knowing this is a personal value, you may plan a trip to Peru to hike Machu Picchu. You can meet the goal of traveling to Peru, and it may be satisfying, but when it is over you'll still be drawn to adventure. Goals can be achieved; values remain even after we achieve a particular goal. Or you may value learning. Your goal may be to get a college degree, but when you've accomplished that goal the value of learning remains. You find yourself learning about all sorts of things that interest you as you go about your life. And when you're learning, you feel alive.

So what happens when you don't achieve your goals? When you rest in the underlying values, it isn't the end of the world. For example, maybe you had financial difficulty and you had to drop out of college. That would be disappointing to be sure, but you can continue to learn. You read books about topics you are interested in. You visit museums, watch YouTube videos, and talk to experts. As long as you are still learning your life has meaning. Our values are not dependent on whether we achieve our goals. Nor is our happiness. As long as we are living our lives in accord with what is meaningful for us—our values—our life feels worth living.

We are happiest when we use our values to choose our goals and our behavior. As long as our goals are in accord with what really matters, our personal values, we are likely to have a satisfying life.

Values versus Social Norms

Another area that often causes confusion around values is social norms, or the expectations of others. Where social norms—those things our society says are important—come from the outside, our personal values come from the inside. Some social norms, like honesty, integrity, kindness, and compassion, for example, are recipes for good relationships. We'd be wise to value them, but the degree to which any individual values them is likely to vary.

We can find ourselves chasing ideals that others tell us are important while neglecting what we ourselves value—for example, chasing financial success by staying in a job that feels boring and confining when your heart longs to create art. It doesn't mean we have to throw caution to the wind and become homeless in the pursuit of creating art. It just means that we have to make room for what makes life worth living. Maybe in this case it simply means taking an art class on the weekends. Or maybe it means becoming a potter and selling pottery for a living. We can consider social norms, but when it comes down to the heart of things we need to know and make room for our personal values.

Most of us have many values. That's why it's important that we know which values rise to the top of the list for us. We call those values our *core values*. They are the strongest values we have or the ones that most matter to us. The ones that make us feel life is worth living.

Values Are the Deepest Thing

Between the confusion around needs, goals, and social norms, sometimes it is hard to identify our personal core values. We may find ourselves stuck on the surface of things. Our values are the deepest thing, so one thing that can help is to keep asking yourself how you would feel if you accomplished what seems like a value. This can help clarify and deepen what is truly a core value for you. For example, if your value seems like financial success, you can ask yourself, "If I was financially successful, how would my life change?" You might find the answer is "I won't have to be so concerned about pleasing others—I'd feel more free to be who I am." (You likely value freedom or authenticity.) Or maybe it would be "Others would want to be with me and look to me for advice. (You likely value connection or wisdom.) Keep asking these clarifying and deepening questions until there isn't a deeper answer. Soon I'll offer you an exercise to help you discover what you truly value.

Personal Core Values and Relational Core Values

In addition to personal core values, we also have qualities or values that are deeply meaningful to us in relationships. These are things that bring the relationship alive for us. These things might be the same as your personal core values, like travel and adventure, or they might be different. They key is to know what makes the relationship a healthy and happy place for you. Some couples find that their relationships go best when they travel and explore together; others find qualities like valuing family, or humor and playfulness, important. And, of course, there are also values like honesty, kindness, and authenticity that often are core to a happy relationship.

Values in Three Directions: Me, You, and We

Looking at this through the lens of our relationships, we see that there are three components to living in accord with our values. We need to know and honor our own values, our partners' values, and those values that benefit our relationships. Since we've already been talking about finding our personal core values and our personal relationship values, let's start with finding your own values.

Finding Your Own Core Values

One way to find out what you value is to work in reverse. In this practice, we'll also take a look at our core relational values as we do in the Compassion for Couples (CFC) course. Let's try that now.

TRY THIS

Discovering Your Core Values

Audio Track 21

Because there are many parts to this exercise, you may find it easier to follow it as a written reflection exercise. Accordingly, you may want to have a pen and paper or journal nearby.

Now, if it feels okay, please close your eyes and, in your mind's eye, find yourself in the room. If you can, smile at yourself in welcome.

If you like, you might place your hand over your heart or elsewhere and feel your body. Your body has been supporting you all your life.

Imagine that you are in your later years. You're sitting in a lovely garden with your partner as you contemplate your life. Looking back to the time between now and then, you feel a deep sense of satisfaction, joy, and contentment. Even though life hasn't always been easy, you managed to stay true to yourself and your relationship to the best of your ability.

Or if you prefer, just let yourself dream of the life you want and long for.

Which core values are represented in that life? For example, adventure, tranquility, financial stability, physical health, compassion, loyalty, pleasure, meaningful work? Please see what it is for you. How did you stay true to yourself?

When you find one you might ask yourself, "If I had that, how would my life change?" to see if there are deeper values underneath.

When you've found the deepest things, these are your personal core values. It may help to write them down.

Now consider which values you embodied that gave you *and* your relationship meaning and satisfaction. In other words, what core values were expressed in your relationship? These can be things like adventure and healthy lifestyle or things like loyalty and compassion. The point is that the presence of these qualities in your relationship led to a satisfying relationship. If you can, stay focused on what you gave rather than what you received. These are your core relational values. You may want to write them down too.

How did your ability to live those core values manifest in your partner? Your relationship? In other words, what effect did living by those core values have? Feel free to make notes on this as well.

What did you discover about what is meaningful to you? What are the similarities and differences in your personal values and your relational values? Is there anything surprising to you? You may want to note which are personal core values and which are relational core values.

Living a self-compassionate life means living in accord with the personal and relational values that are important to you.

Considering Your Partner's Values

For most of us, the biggest obstacle to knowing our partners' core values is that we don't see them as separate people with their own preferred way of being in the world. We are trying to get them over to the way we think they should be in the world. Taking a step back and considering our partners through their eyes can create precious space for both people.

Do you know what your partner's values are? What makes your partner happy? What does your partner value in the relationship? When I do the following core values exercise with couples in the CFC program, I find that people are often surprised at how well their partners know them. Of course sometimes they are surprised that their partners don't know them well. Either way, it's great to check this out as best you can. If you're one of the lucky ones who is reading this book with a partner, this should be easy. Your partner will actually do the exercise too and then you can share your answers with each other. If not, there are two ways to approach this: discussing and observing.

TRY THIS
Discussing Your Partner's Core Values

If it feels right, you can have a casual conversation over dinner or at another relaxed time about what really makes your partner's life complete. Or find out what your partner imagines would make it complete. You don't have to drill your partner or even let your partner know you are trying to uncover her core values. You can simply be curious. You may want to ask things like:

- What was the happiest time in your life? What made that such a wonderful time for you?

- If you could do anything right now, what would it be? What would make that attractive right now?

- At the end of your life, what would you be proud of having accomplished?

- If you could live your life over again, what changes would you make?

As you listen to the answers, see if you can identify the theme that runs through them. Let yourself see your partner through your partner's eyes rather than your own. Remember that this is about seeing and understanding your partner more clearly.

TRY THIS

Observing Your Partner's Core Values

Your partner may not be comfortable having such a conversation, and that's okay. By observing what your partner is "living for" you can also discover his core values. For example, how does your partner spend his time? Sometimes just how a person allocates his time can give a clue to what they value. Lots of time with family? Friends? Playing? Working? Exercising? Healthy eating?

The trouble is that we don't always allocate our time to what is important to us, so you need to also observe what actually makes your partner happy. For example, when your partner spends time with family, does it light him up? Does your partner look happier than before gathering with family? Or does it appear to exhaust and deplete him? This will give you a clue about whether your partner values spending time with family or is doing so out of a sense of duty and obligation. Does your partner love to travel and explore? Is your partner always up for the next adventure, or does he prefer to stay home and tend the garden? Does your partner love things that give him a sense of freedom, or does your partner like things that are predictable and routine? What makes him happy? You might also consider what is a personal core value for your partner and what his relational core values may be.

What Did You Learn about Your Partner's Core Values?

- If you both did the "Discovering Your Core Values" exercise on page 178, please take some time to share what you found with each other.

- If your partner didn't do the exercise, but you were able to have the discussion suggested on page 180 with her, what did you learn about her core values?

- If your partner wasn't available to discuss their values with you, what did you discover by observing her?

When you feel you have a sense of your partner's personal core values and their relational values (either through discussion or observation), it is helpful to write those down too.

In the next exercise you'll have a chance to use these to discover your shared relationship values.

The foundation for intimacy is knowing what makes life meaningful for the other person—what they value and who they are.

When we know someone well or when we open our eyes and look for clues about the nature of another person, we begin to have a sense of who that person is. We understand what makes life meaningful for that person. Knowing who they are and what they value is the foundation for intimacy.

Finding Shared Relationship Values

Beyond tending to the needs of each individual partner, the relationship itself needs proper care and feeding. Of course what the relationship needs is informed by what each of you values. Just as you used discussion and/or observation to uncover what your partner's core values are, you can use the same tools to uncover what the relationship needs.

TRY THIS

Talking About What You Discovered

If you're both reading this book and have done the Discovering Your Core Values exercise, you simply need to come together and take turns telling your partner (and listening to your partner) what you discovered about your own personal and relationship values. It's helpful to have a piece of paper where you list your respective values as you share them. (Please don't worry if your partner didn't do the exercise; below we will use discussing and observing to get to the same place.)

Once you have seen and heard each other, you can turn your attention to looking at your shared values. Often people find things in common on their individual lists, like family, travel, or authenticity. They know that these are then core to the relationship. When you find these shared values, write them in a separate column about what the relationship needs. If you don't have overlaps on your lists, you can ask each other what it is that makes your relationship go well. Maybe you find that relaxing together has a positive effect. Or perhaps things tend to go well when you explore new places. Maybe you like to learn together or spend time with family. These should also go on the relationship values list.

One very common thing that happens is that couples look at their lists and see a lot of differences. This can feel really disturbing, especially if the values appear to be incompatible. Maybe one partner values freedom and the other values connection. Each can feel a bit freaked out by the other's value. In reality, when partners understand and support each other's values, these can be worked with without too much difficulty. Maybe the partner who values freedom goes skydiving with her partner's blessing because that feels really freeing and her partner cares about her happiness. Then, knowing how important connection is to the other partner, the skydiving partner makes it a point to come home and tell her partner all about the experience, while also asking about her partner's day. In this way these values actually *support* the relationship. Having experiences beyond the relationship can enliven and enrich the relationship when they are brought back into the relationship and shared. The value of freedom helps the relationship grow, and the value of connection helps anchor it in safety and reliability. So, not to worry if your values appear different. Get creative in how you might honor them in a way that strengthens your relationship.

Managing Different Values: Michael and Stephanie

Michael and Stephanie were at a crossroads of sorts. Michael, the sole provider for their family, was expecting a layoff at work. Although this was anxiety provoking for him, he saw it as an opportunity to launch his own business. He valued professional success and saw that as running his own business. He also valued being a good provider for his family and thought the best way to accomplish that would be to go out on his own. He knew it was risky, but he believed that the bigger the risk, the bigger the reward. A big reward was important to him.

His wife, Stephanie, also valued Michael supporting the family. However, she valued financial stability far more than accumulating wealth. She was willing to live a more modest, but still comfortable, life with the security of Michael having a regular paycheck and benefits. She really wanted him to focus on finding a new employer should the layoff happen.

At first, as they discussed what to do they really butted heads. He pushed for launching his own business and she for finding a new job. As they each argued their position, both felt unseen and unimportant to the other, and the distress was escalating on both sides. It was only when they slowed down long enough to consider their deeper motivations—and why those mattered—that they could come to a solution that served them both.

With the help of their therapist, for a moment they let go of focusing on outcome and became curious about why each position was important. When Michael explained that he valued financial success because it made him feel more powerful and less subject to having to please others (his boss and coworkers), Stephanie understood that the professional autonomy that came with starting his own business was a deeply held value for Michael. She could see how it related to his having had a domineering father. She loved him and wanted to support something so meaningful for him.

When Stephanie explained that she valued financial stability because while her own family was taking risks on their way to financial success, they sometimes relied on her to provide money she made from babysitting so that they had enough food to eat. This had been really scary for her. Michael could see that for Stephanie being a good provider had more to do with providing financial security than accumulating wealth. He didn't want her to feel the constant insecurity and fear she'd had when growing up, and he was motivated to find a way to make her feel more financially secure.

Once they understood what the other valued and why those values were meaningful, their hearts opened a bit to each other. Michael was now investing in Stephanie's feeling safe, and Stephanie was invested in Michael's feeling successful. Still unwilling to give up their own needs and values, they began to be curious about how they might find a solution that met both of their needs. How could Michael pursue the professional autonomy he valued while also honoring the financial security that Stephanie valued? They put their heads together and began forming a business plan. They looked at how much savings they had and how long that would last. They looked at how long it would be before Michael's business would be able to support them. In the end they decided he should give it a try, but they also had clearly agreed how they would know if and when it was time for him to find a new employer. Michael felt supported in launching his new business, and Stephanie felt reassured that it would happen in a way that wouldn't threaten their financial security. Rather than pushing them farther apart, as it had in the beginning when they were each battling for the outcome they wanted, the process of exploring, *and honoring*, each person's values actually brought them closer together. It turned out their values were indeed different, but not incompatible, as they'd first believed.

TRY THIS
Talking About the Relationship

Most people won't have a partner who is also reading the book. That's okay too. You've already done the work of creating your own list of core values and also uncovering your partner's core values. You can write those down on a sheet of paper as I've suggested above. Then look for values that overlap. These are likely to be shared relational values. When these values are honored in your relationship, the relationship grows stronger. You can augment this list by being curious with your partner about what makes your relationship stronger. You might ask questions like:

- What is your favorite memory of us?
- When did you know we were right for each other?
- What is the healthiest (or best) thing about our relationship?
- If one of us was suddenly gone, what would you miss the most about our relationship?

Questions like these can also help you identify what makes your relationship stronger and healthier.

TRY THIS
Observing the Relationship

If you're someone whose partner isn't comfortable with such discussions, observation may be your best route. You might consider your own answers to the questions above. Then consider how you think your partner might answer when you look through their eyes. Make it an experiment; try to be true to some of those relational values and observe the effects. Is there more life in the relationship when you do?

Whether you use discussion or observation to uncover your shared relational values, making a list of what the relationship needs can give you a road map to the proper care and feeding of *your* relationship. Once you have that road map, you can decide on goals that may support what your relationship needs. For example, making a plan to travel can feed the core value of adventure, or planning a date night schedule can feed the core value of connection. Have some fun exploring how this new road map may guide you to a deeper and more satisfying relationship.

Honoring Our Core Values

As with everything in this book, intention and tone matter a great deal. We don't want to use what we discover as a weapon against our partners: "You know freedom is important to me, and you aren't honoring me!!!" Rather, we want to learn what is deeply important here as a way of cultivating wisdom and compassion. When we know what our needs, our partners' needs, and our relational needs are, it's like having a road map toward a more satisfying life.

We can use this map to honor our own values and needs. When we see and speak up about what matters to us, we are bringing our vulnerable selves into the relationship and risking being seen. There is no intimacy without vulnerability. To be seen by your partner, you must first see and honor yourself. Knowing what brings you alive can motivate you to tend to your own happiness, rather than stewing in frustration because your partner isn't on the same page. You can root yourself in what really matters to you. Explaining what you are living for can help your partner really see you and want to support you. Because underneath everything, most likely your partner really cares about your well-being.

At the same time, we need to make space to see and understand our partners at a deep level. What does your partner value? What is your partner living for? And, when we remember that we care about *their* well-being, along with our own, we are motivated to find a way to support their having what they need too. There is actually a joy in knowing something meaningful is happening for them. And in the words of Maya Angelou, "I've learned that people will forget what you said, people will forget what you did, but people will never forget how *you made them feel*." When you see and support your partner's deepest values, your partner feels safe, supported, and truly loved. Nothing says "You matter to me" more than feeling supported in our deepest desires. Who doesn't want to feel their partner is rooting for them?

Sometimes we can show up for each person, but in the busyness of life we forget about what the relationship needs. When this happens, couples grow apart—even when each individual is growing. If you find this is happening in your relationship, it's even more important to focus on your shared relationship values. What is it or what was it that brought that spark of life and delight into your relationship? Time to figure out how to begin including that again.

Maybe you used to take exotic vacations together, but now you have a family and are short on time and money, so an exotic vacation is out of the question right now. You can ask yourself, "What value did that vacation satisfy?" Was it time alone together? A sense of exploring something new? Something else? If it was time alone together, you might commit to a "date night" once a week—even if it is in the dining room at home with the kids in the other room watching a movie. Or if it was more about exploring something new, maybe finding new places to explore as a family begins to meet that need for adventure.

The point is that it is easy to let the obstacles in life take over and find yourself drifting with those currents like a rudderless boat. You may not be heading in the direction you want to go. But if you can land in and identify what brings meaning and well-being into your relationship, then, like using the rudder, you can use that knowledge to steer your relationship back toward healthier waters. When we anchor ourselves in our core relational values, there is a sense of "I'm rooting for us!"

10

"How Can We Really Get Each Other?"

Using Compassionate Communication Skills

> The roots of a lasting relationship are mindfulness, deep listening, and loving speech, and a strong community to support you.
>
> —THICH NHAT HANH

Communication is the method we use to understand each other. In any given moment when we really "get" each other, the heart opens. That's why compassionate communication is so important. Without intentionally cultivating compassion as the basis for communication we often end up communicating from the threat/defense or drive systems.

Many of us know some sort of formula for communication. One I like is the formula from the *nonviolent communication* program: I feel _____ when you _____ and I need _____. It's a great formula for many reasons. It is designed to take us out of blaming mode and put us in the more vulnerable mode of sharing how we feel and what we need. When you're in this more vulnerable mode, it is easier for your partner to hear you. It's like a cartoon of two porcupines I saw a long time ago. Two porcupines are standing side by side, one with its quills lying down and the other with its quills sticking out.

The porcupine with its quills out is saying to the one with its quills down, "Why don't you ever want to cuddle anymore?" Vulnerability helps you put your quills down so that your partner can come closer without getting poked. It also gives the listener a road map for how to be successful in the relationship when you say directly what you need. I can't tell you how much partners appreciate explicit directions on what to do. So many times they want to help and are distressed when their partner is in pain—and they are afraid of being unsuccessful. It is such a relief to know what their partner would actually find helpful.

Here's the question, though: Do formulas like this always work? Not really. Imagine that your partner does that annoying thing he always does—the one that you're really sick of. Let's say your partner is late again, leaving you sitting alone in a restaurant or home alone with hungry kids and a dog that needs to be walked. Imagine that you've been sitting there waiting for your partner for 5, then 10, then 20, then 35 minutes, all the while going over in your mind how insensitive your partner is and how alone you are. By the time your partner walks in the door 45 minutes late you're pretty steamed. At that point are you really able to follow the formula? Probably not. Your system isn't wired for communication. You're in the threat/defense system where you're wired for fighting or fleeing.

But let's say you've been studying how to communicate and working really hard at having a better relationship. So remarkably, even though you're in your threat/defense system, you remember the formula and squelch the urge to blast your partner. Instead, you say something like "I feel angry when you're late and I need to know I can count on you to show up when you say you will." You used the right words, but if you were still angry and full of blame or disgust, the message you sent was likely still one of anger, blame, or disgust.

It's More about the State We Are in Than the Words We Use

So much of our communication happens beyond the words and even the tone of voice we use. The nonverbal cues we give count much more than what we verbalize. Our state is what gets communicated, whether it's what we want to communicate or not. Consider these three scenarios:

Scenario 1: You've had a great night's sleep. You wake up naturally, feeling good and ready to be awake. You look over at your partner and you're happy to see her. You're feeling really good about yourself, your partner, and your relationship, and you're looking forward to the day ahead. You greet your partner with the words "Good morning."

Scenario 2: You wake up to the alarm. You feel terrible. You've hardly gotten any sleep, and you have a day ahead of you that you are dreading. To make matters worse, you look over at your partner and remember how irritated you are with him. The day is off to a terrible start for you. You greet your partner with the words "Good morning."

Scenario 3: You wake up feeling good. You look over and see your partner, and you feel really good about them and your relationship. You notice how attracted you are to them and you feel like flirting in hopes the morning will get even better. You greet your partner with the words "Good morning."

In each scenario you've used the same words, but what you communicated was very different because of the differing states you were in. In the first scenario what was communicated was that you were happy to see your partner. The second communicated that you weren't happy to see your partner, and the third sent the message that you were interested in being intimate. Because we catch each other's emotions, your partner was able to understand what you were really communicating, even though the actual words were "Good morning." It's that "emotion contagion" we talked about in Chapter 3, which is not always helpful. When we are upset, we don't really want our partner to catch our upset. We want to feel that our partner feels and understands our pain, but even more we are hoping that their understanding will open their heart and they will comfort and soothe us.

Take the case of Brian and Tai. Brian had been home with the kids all day. It had been a busy day and there was the mess of having small kids, but he was feeling really happy. It was satisfying to be home with them, and he found himself feeling grateful to be able to be with them. Tai had a terrible day at work. He lost a patient and had a conflict with a coworker. He was still wound up from the stress of the day when he arrived home. He was hoping for a peaceful environment in which he could recover from the stress of the day. When he walked in and saw the kids' toys everywhere, it all came to a head and he was furious.

He stopped himself from saying what he really wanted to say: "All you have to do is look after the kids and keep the house tidy, Brian, and you can't even do that!" He knew he needed to send a kinder message, so instead he managed to say, "I really need to come home to a tidy home." But his face was red, the veins in his forehead were popping out, and his voice was raised. Brian felt the anger behind the comment and instantly became angry too. He found himself snapping back, "I guess you don't even care that I've worked all day taking care of our kids and making sure they grow up feeling loved. I don't really matter to you, do I?" Now both partners were angry and Tai felt even worse. What he really wanted was for Brian to understand that he'd had a hard day and offer him some support. He wanted compassion.

From Emotion Contagion to Compassion

Tania Singer, a researcher who studies empathy and compassion, talks about the difference between emotion contagion, empathy, and compassion and how they build on each other.

Emotion Contagion

Emotion contagion is at the root of things. We feel what others are feeling. We catch their emotion, as in the story I told in Chapter 3 about how I found myself laughing, even though I didn't find the balloon funny the way my children did, or the story of Brian and Tai above. This ability to feel what those around us are feeling is really helpful. It connects us to others and helps us notice the state they are in. For most of us, shared laughter is much more powerful than laughing by ourselves. Unfortunately, shared anger is more powerful too.

Empathy

A step up from emotion contagion, Singer notes, is empathy. She defines empathy as emotion contagion plus the sense of a separate self. For example, I feel your sadness, but I know it is your sadness I am feeling rather than my own. This sense of sorting out whose emotions are whose is really helpful in communication. We don't have to catch the emotions ourselves. We can use the feeling of emotion contagion to help us understand how the other person is feeling. It even works if the other person doesn't yet know how they are feeling or have words to describe what they are feeling. As a therapist, I find this really help-ful. A patient who comes in feeling sad doesn't actually want me to become sad. If I did, they'd feel like they needed to take care of me. Rather, they want me to know and feel their sadness without catching it myself. That way I can remain stable and help them. In fact, this space to discern who is feeling what gives us the space to respond rather than react.

Tai didn't really want Brian to become angry. He wanted Brian to notice that Tai was angry—*as a sign Tai was in distress.* And rather than catch the anger, he hoped Brian would care that he was in dis-tress and offer him the space he needed to calm and care for himself.

Compassion

A step up from empathy, according to Singer, is compassion. She defines compassion as empathy plus love. When my patients are sad, for example, they don't just want me to know and accept that they are sad. They also want to know that I care about them. Their sadness matters to me because they matter to me. And that love part (the fact that I do care about them) is protective for me, too.

People often wonder how I'm able to listen to people's pain all day. (It seems that's what they think therapists do.) When they won-der about that, they're really assuming emotion contagion—that I would also be in pain all day. Or at least empathy—that I'd be feeling people's pain all day even if I knew it wasn't mine. What they don't know is that when there is a strong sense of caring about another per-son we can hold the pain without becoming overwhelmed. Then the dominant feeling in the end is love or care. That love is the buffer that can hold the pain without our burning out. When the love is stronger than the pain, the predominant feeling is love. Being in a state of caring about someone else is not depleting in the way that just resonating with someone's pain is.

In our romantic relationships everything is amplified because the other person is so important to us. So when things go wrong, it feels like an emergency. We can't lose this person who is at the core of our lives. When we are feeling the threat of that loss, we are cut off from the care that could allow us to move into a state of compassion. We either stay stuck in the threat/defense system or recruit the drive system in hopes of fixing the problem.

Brian and Tai each felt the threat of losing the other. When Tai snapped at Brian, Brian felt the loss of the usually kind and supportive partner Tai was. Brian felt threatened by that loss, and he also caught Tai's anger. Now Brian was in his threat/defense system and snapped at Tai to protest the loss. When Brian snapped at him, Tai lost the one person he could usually count on for support. Now both were in their threat/defense systems and a downward relational spiral was under way. One or both of them would need to pause and land in compassion before they could turn the spiral around.

The thing we miss is that the problem isn't the problem. In Brian and Tai's case, the problem wasn't the toys on the floor, as Tai suggested. The problem was that Tai was stressed and needed care. Problems—even unsolvable ones— are a normal part of life, even though we find them unpleasant at best. In fact, relationship expert John Gottman's research suggests that 69 percent of problems in a relationship are unsolvable. The problem is that we don't remember to activate our care system when we are distressed. So when we communicate, we aren't really communicating love and care—we are communicating whatever state we are in:

> The "problem" isn't the problem. The problem is not remembering to shift into the care system when distressed.

Threat/defense system:

- "It's your fault" gets communicated when we're in fight mode.
- "I don't want to be here" gets communicated when we're in flight mode.
- "I don't feel safe being vulnerable with you" gets communicated when we're in freeze mode.

Drive system:

- "You can't handle things" gets communicated when we're in control mode.
- "There's something wrong with you" gets communicated when we're in criticize mode.
- "You're broken" or "You're incapable" gets communicated when we're in fix mode.

> Love is the buffer that allows us to hold the problems we're struggling with and not go into a downward relational spiral.

What we really want and need when we are distressed is to be loved. Love can be the buffer that makes it possible to hold the problems we, our partner, and our relationship have—without moving into a downward relational spiral.

Moving into Compassionate Communication

So how do Brian and Tai—and the rest of us—pause and land in compassion? We can tap the three components of self-compassion: mindfulness, common humanity, and kindness. Or, as I like to think of them, loving (kindness), connected (common humanity) presence (mindfulness).

Mindfulness (presence): We need to notice how we are feeling and how our partners are feeling. We allow ourselves and our partners to be just as they are. And we discern whose feelings these are and what is happening here. Brian might have noticed anger arising in him. If he paused and acknowledged his anger, then realized that he was actually happy, he might have recognized that it was Tai's anger that he was feeling. This may have cued him in to the fact that Tai was in distress. It may also have given Brian a bit of space where Tai's anger no longer had such a grip on him, even though it was unpleasant.

Common humanity (connected): We remember that "just like me" my partner wants to be happy and free of suffering. Just like me, my partner doesn't always put her best foot forward, especially when scared or sad. Just like me, my partner also wants to feel loved and accepted and is doing her best to show up in this relationship even when it isn't going well. It would have been helpful if rather than judging Tai as selfish or uncaring for his angry outburst, Brian landed in the understanding that he too isn't at his best when he is distressed. That sometimes when Brian is angry he lashes out when what he really needs is to be loved through his difficulty—like the porcupine with its quills out that longs to be cuddled. Brian could say to himself, "Just like me, Tai gets angry when he doesn't feel safe."

Kindness (loving): We remember this is someone we love and for whom we wish happiness and freedom from suffering. We allow our hearts to open and drop our defensive behavior. We allow feelings of compassion for ourselves and our partners to arise, and we turn our attention and thoughts toward actions that reflect our desire to help this person. Kindness is applied with wisdom when we consider what would actually be skillful, which may not always be in line with our reactions.

Knowing that Tai is distressed and being able to use Brian's own past experiences with anger when he is distressed, and remembering how much Tai means to him, Brian would likely have the impulse to identify and offer whatever Tai might need right now. From this softened place and in touch with how much he cares about Tai, perhaps he might have said something like "Wow, you sound really angry. I take it you had a really hard time at work today. Do you want to talk about it, or would you just like some space? I'm here for you; just let me know what you need." And beyond the particular words, a loving presence would have come through. Just by activating his own care system through the practice of mindfulness, common humanity, and kindness, Brian may have changed the downward relational spiral into an upward relational spiral.

The chart below gives a sense of the stages of compassion and the skills and actions that are needed to meet each other with compassion, even in difficult times.

Meeting Each Other with Compassion

Stage	Skill	Action
When we open to each other as we are	Mindfulness	Accept
Understanding our shared human condition	Common humanity	Connect
With wishes of well-being	Loving-kindness	Love
Even in painful times	Compassion	Comfort

This takes some practice. It isn't possible to connect deeply with our partners without also knowing our own vulnerability. We need to risk being vulnerable to open to the possibility of connection.

In *The Book of Awakening: Having the Life You Want by Being Present to the Life You Have*, Mark Nepo beautifully illustrates this point:

We waste so much energy trying to cover up who we are, when beneath every attitude is the want to be loved, and beneath every anger is a wound to be healed, and beneath every sadness is the fear that there will not be enough time.

When we hesitate in being direct, we unknowingly slip something on, some added layer of protection that keeps us from feeling the world, and often that thin covering is the beginning of a loneliness which, if not put down, diminishes our chances of joy.

It's like wearing gloves every time we touch something, and then, forgetting we chose to put them on, we complain that nothing feels quite real. In this way, our challenge each day is not to get dressed to face the world, but to unglove ourselves so that the doorknob feels cold, and the car handle feels wet, and the kiss good-bye feels like the lips of another being, soft and unrepeatable.

However, even when we're vulnerable, our partners, just like us, are human and won't always respond in the way we find helpful. This is where our self-compassion practice is so very helpful. We can risk closeness *and* pain because we can comfort and soothe ourselves . . . and our partners.

Blocks to Compassionate Communication

When we aren't feeling comfortable being vulnerable with our partners, we can fall into habits that really interfere with compassionate communication. One of these habits is criticism.

Why Do We Criticize?

Criticism is a common block to compassionate communication. When being vulnerable doesn't feel safe, we can use criticism in an attempt to make ourselves and our relationships safer, even though it typically makes the relationship more unsafe. When I ask participants in the CFC program why we criticize, they say things like:

- So my partner stops doing those things that need to change and I can feel safe being close to them.
- It's a defense mechanism so I don't feel like the worst person in the room.
- So my partner will do things the way I like them and I'll feel comfortable.
- To help my partner become their best self so I can be proud of them.

The theme that runs through these answers is that we are trying to keep ourselves, our partners, and our relationships safe—all the while protecting ourselves from being too vulnerable. So we shine the spotlight on our partners and let them know they should do things differently. We want them to be vulnerable and to take on the vulnerable work of changing while we keep ourselves hidden from view. However, without allowing ourselves to be seen, we never quite feel loved.

In some ways, criticism can actually be a bid for connection. We're trying to make the conditions safer so we can be vulnerable. We can also think of criticism as a kind of protest. "You haven't been hearing me when my emotional volume was at a 5. What happens if I turn it up to a 10? Are you hearing how important it is to me now that I'm yelling and pointing my finger at you?" Sadly, the answer is usually no. We don't hear very well when we are under attack. Criticism may be common and understandable, but it doesn't actually make the relationship safer. It doesn't bring us closer. It usually pushes our partners farther away.

Why Do We Withdraw or Avoid?

Withdrawing is another strategy we often use when we aren't feeling safe. When I ask participants in the CFC course why we withdraw or avoid, they say things like:

- I'm afraid if I stay I'll get hurt.
- I'm afraid if I stay I'll say or do something to hurt my partner.
- I'm triggered, and I need some space to calm down.
- I don't know how to talk about my feelings; it's really uncomfortable for me.
- I can see the argument isn't going anywhere, and I don't want it to get worse.

The theme that runs through these answers also has to do with keeping ourselves, our partners, and our relationships safe. We are trying to avoid conflict and the damage it can do to our relationships. We don't want to be hurt, and we don't want to hurt our partners.

However, withdrawing leaves your partner all alone, where your partner is likely to feel unloved. Love flows where attention goes. No attention equals no love. This doesn't mean that we can't take a break.

In fact, it is skillful to take a break and give ourselves what we need so that we can come from a place of responsiveness rather than reactivity. There is a difference between taking a break in the service of avoidance or resistance and taking a break in the service of compassion.

What we do when we take a break matters. Do you put things out of your mind by turning to distractions like Netflix or your favorite hobby without a plan to come back and deal with the issues? If so, that's avoidance. Or do you take a break to soothe yourself and figure out how best to come back and discuss the issues? If so, that's likely compassion in action. Even if your intention is compassion, however, you need to consider what your partner needs as you take your break. It makes a big difference if you can say something reassuring as you take a break, like "I'm too triggered and can't communicate well right now. I'm going to take a break and calm myself by going for a walk so things don't get worse. I love you, and I'll come back and talk to you about it when I get back from my walk." The key is that your partner understand the intention behind the break and that you are coming back. Then they can feel reassured that they are important to you rather than feeling unloved and abandoned.

Steps to Staying Connected with Compassion

When strong emotions arise in us, they often drive our behavior and harm our relationships if we let them. We find ourselves acting out of fear, anger, desperation, shame. When we allow our reactivity to run the show, we lose touch with our own vulnerability, the vulnerability of the other person, and our ability to respond from a place of wisdom and compassion. Whenever our suffering exceeds our resources, unskillful behavior is often the result.

The work you've done in Parts I and II of this book, as well as your work on core values in the preceding chapter, were all laying the foundation for putting compassion into action. Keep practicing those. The stronger the foundation we build, the better we weather the storms of difficulty.

When those storms do hit, we really need each other. We need to turn toward, rather than away from, our partner. To do that we need to make communication safe. We can learn to speak and listen from a place of loving, connected presence. We can meet ourselves and each other with compassion.

To move from a place of reactivity to responding with compassion, there are four basic steps:

1. *We need to disengage from reactivity.* We begin by giving ourselves space after noticing we are caught in reactivity. We pause and anchor ourselves in the sensation of the breath or other sensations and create the possibility of a more stable awareness. This is the practice of mindfulness.

2. *We turn our attention to our own state of being.* What is it that was triggered in us, and what is it that we need? Can we choose to respond to ourselves with wisdom and compassion? In doing so, we awaken the possibility of opening to others. This is the practice of self-compassion.

3. *We turn our attention to the vulnerability of the other person.* Is it possible that we don't know the other's full story or experience? We begin to tend to them by skillfully listening to what they are saying. Then we broaden our observations to take in the person as a whole. When we open to the experience and vulnerability of the other person, we allow our hearts to melt in response to them. This is the practice of compassion.

4. *We turn our attention toward choosing our response.* We remind ourselves of our values, and we choose to respond in a way that has integrity for us. Our response is then rooted in both wisdom and compassion. Here we are guided by our values.

I've put all these steps together to help make speaking and listening with compassion easier.

Finding Your Compassionate Voice: Speaking with Compassion

One of my favorite practices is one I developed based on the STOP practice you learned in Chapter 6. We tend to ourselves with STOP, and when our physiology has settled, we turn our attention to our partner with LOVE. Let's try that now.

STOP and LOVE

Audio Track 22

Begin by finding a comfortable position.

Allow your eyes to close if that is comfortable for you and bring your attention inside.

Find a sense of yourself in the room and offer yourself a smile of welcome.

Please call to mind a time when you and your partner were having a disagreement and you found yourself a bit distressed—not the worst fight you ever had and nothing traumatic. Just choose something distressing enough that you feel it in the body. A 3–4 on the scale of distress. Even though you might be tempted to work with something difficult here, you'll be more likely to be successful if you stick with a 3–4.

Or you can call to mind something you want to tell your partner that is difficult for you to talk about. Remember, this is an opportunity to practice and build skill, so please don't choose something that is the most difficult thing to discuss; stick with a 3–4. Maybe you're really tired of eating at that restaurant your partner loves to go to. Or maybe you've been doing more of the cooking than you like. Maybe you would like to take up a new hobby that you are afraid your partner won't approve of.

This takes some time. When you have something in mind, take a moment to write it down briefly. Then let yourself open to the situation, feeling your desire for something different.

To tend to ourselves we begin with the STOP practice:

S—Stop. Remember to pause. We begin breaking through reactivity by slowing down, pausing, and making space for something new to happen. Let go of the story and turn your attention toward this moment.

T—Take a breath. Actually, take a few breaths. Let everything else rest in the background as you privilege your awareness on the sensation of breathing. Just breathing. Where do you feel the breath? What does it feel like? Notice the sensations wherever you feel them most easily.

Anchoring our awareness in the breath gives us the chance to anchor in this moment and this body. Feel free to use a different anchor for awareness if the breath isn't the right anchor for you. For example, you might feel your feet or hands.

O—Observe. What is happening here in this moment and this body? Notice the thoughts, emotions, and sensations present. No need to change them in any way. Just notice them.

Allow the attention to broaden a bit to fully take in what is happening right now. Given your new perspective, perhaps ask yourself, "What do I need right now?"

P—Proceed to practice. Now that you have a better understanding of what is happening and what you need, see if you can find a way to honor your needs. Perhaps STOP was all you needed. Or maybe you need to take a walk, have tea, or sit in meditation. Maybe there are some words you need to hear. Can you say them to yourself now?

The point is to give ourselves what we need to move out of the state of reactivity and into a state of responsiveness. Tending to our true needs rather than reacting from whatever place was triggered in us is the key.

See where you are right now. You can stay right here if you need to. No need to move on if you still need soothing.

If you are in a state of responsiveness, you can turn your attention to the vulnerability of the other person with LOVE.

To tend to our partners and relationships we continue with the LOVE practice:

L—Listen. This means letting go of ourselves, our vision of how things are or should be, our being right or wrong, good or bad. Let these things rest in the background.

Listen to what the other person is saying. What is their perspective, their truth? What is it they want us to know? Or if you haven't yet had a conversation about it, how might they feel? What might they say?

When we truly open to taking in what the other is saying, we allow ourselves to be touched and moved, to learn things we didn't know. Listening is both an act of generosity and an act of love.

O—Observe. Taking in the other's experience requires more than just hearing the words they are saying. What is the tone of the words? What does the body look like? Are there tears? A hot red face? A look of fear?

As we listen to this person, we might notice the state they are in. Do they seem scared, angry, lonely, or sad? Is their behavior reflective of their efforts to be safe and loved? Is there something underneath their possible reactivity? Are they just trying to keep themselves safe?

If we know them well, we might also know this to be a core pain they carry, and we can deepen our understanding of the vulnerable situation they are in. We can remember that, just like us and all beings, this person wishes to be happy and free from suffering.

We allow our hearts to be touched by the state of the other. We see more clearly what the other person needs.

V—Values. It is helpful to pause here, to remember our own core values. Whenever we take in the vulnerability of another, we have a choice in how we will respond to them. Grounding that choice in our core values allows a wise and compassionate response.

It can help to remember that this is someone we love and are loved by. We might remind ourselves of how important it is to us that they feel safe and loved, free from harm. We can remember how we wish all beings to be happy and free from suffering.

We might remember our own values or even vows to be compassionate, courageous, or kind, or whatever they may be.

We pause and ground ourselves in our own values and vows, and then it becomes clearer which actions are in alignment with what is deeply meaningful to us. Grounding in this way allows our response to be guided by wisdom.

E—Express. This is the action part of compassion. When we have deepened our understanding of ourselves and the other person, and allowed wisdom and compassion to arise, it often becomes much easier to know how to respond now.

What do you need to say or not say? Is there a gesture that would be helpful? A smile, eye contact, a pat on the back, or a hug? Perhaps the most compassionate thing you can do is to say no or otherwise set a boundary.

Or maybe it is to remind your partner of their importance to you. Often, letting the other know that we see and value them is the most loving thing we can do. Trust your own response and follow through by expressing whatever is needed right now.

Now write a letter to them, freely and spontaneously practicing what you might want to say to them.

Note: These letters are just for you to practice saying what you would like to say. Later we will practice compassionate listening and compassionate speaking. This letter is a way for you to practice speaking in a way that feels safe.

How did this practice go for you? Was your letter different from the way you would ordinarily speak to your partner? It sometimes feels awkward to slow down so much and go through this process. Over time, however, the process becomes second nature, and you can move through it much more quickly.

Another thing that sometimes arises is that when you think about what you might say to your partner, you might find your physiology activated again and find you are back in the threat/defense system. This just means you need to go back to the STOP practice again—particularly the part where you give yourself what you need. Or it may mean you've taken on too big an issue to begin with. Can you repeat the process with something much less difficult?

If you find yourself *always* triggered when you think of speaking to your partner, beginning these conversations in the safety of couples therapy is likely to be helpful. Good couples therapists interrupt downward spirals and help to restore safety, and a skilled therapist can give on-the-spot coaching and safety so you can feel successful in speaking up.

The Four Cs of Compassionate Speaking

Of course, putting speaking into practice *with* your partner can feel a bit more challenging than practicing by writing a letter. The four Cs of compassionate speaking can help:

1. *Centering: Awake body*—It is helpful to pause here, take a moment to focus your attention on your breathing (or another safe anchor), and come into the body. Release any unnecessary tension.

2. *Curiosity: Open mind*—Noticing what might be under your anger or frustration. Are there vulnerable feelings that need attention? Keep the focus on yourself and speak from vulnerability.

3. *Connection: Warm heart*—Remembering the listener is someone you love and are loved by even when distress arises. Speaking with an attitude of gentleness. Avoiding blame, accusations, and name-calling.

4. *Compassion: Kind action*—Is there something you need from the listener? How might you feel calmed, comforted, reassured? Ask for what you need.

You can always practice the STOP practice or any mindfulness or self-compassion practice that you've found helpful whenever you feel distress on the horizon. When you speak, you should feel free to take your time, to pause whenever you need, and to resume speaking when you know what you want to say.

Cultivating Loving, Connected Presence: Listening with Compassion

Of course, there are two sides to compassionate communication. How we listen makes it safe, or not, for our partners to speak up when something is bothering them. Ideally, we also want to be in our care system.

When we open to another person's pain, especially when it is about us, we can feel overwhelmed and pulled into reactivity. One of the common reactions is to try to fix or advise the other person so that he is no longer in pain and, therefore, we don't "catch" the emotion from him. In other words, we try to get out of our own pain—the pain that comes with empathic resonance—by fixing the other person so there is no more pain to resonate with.

Another common reaction is to distance ourselves by blaming or criticizing. However, listening requires that we let go of our "story" of things and really take in what the other person is saying. What your partner needs when distressed is your presence—your loving, connected presence. So notice the urge to butt in and respond or defend yourself. Instead, practice staying present and as open as you can while your partner is talking. The four Cs of compassionate listening can be helpful here too.

The Four Cs of Compassionate Listening

1. *Centered: Awake body*—It is helpful to pause here, take a moment to focus your attention on your breathing (or another safe anchor) and come into the body. Release any unnecessary tension.

2. *Curious: Open mind*—Try opening the mind. Become a detective, trying to understand what the speaker is communicating. When

it is your turn to speak, you can ask questions to obtain a better understanding. Let go of toxic certainty, remembering it is about them, not you; listening with an attitude of encouragement.

3. *Connected: Warm heart*—Remember the speaker is someone you love and are loved by even when distress arises. Remember a time you felt that way too. "Just like me, this person _____."

4. *Compassionate: Kind action*—Is there anything you can say or do to help calm, comfort, or reassure your partner? "What do you need? How can I help?"

Like anything else, compassionate listening is a skill that can be developed, even if it feels awkward at first. One thing that helps is to approach your conversations with the intention of listening to understand rather than listening to solve the problem. When you focus on process rather than outcome, your partner will be able to feel the difference. When you listen to understand, your partner is likely to feel important and cared about and in the end may feel understood. When you focus on outcome, your partner may feel unimportant to you, that what you really want is just to get whatever outcome you desire. They may come away from the conversation feeling unseen and uncared for. It's a small shift that makes a world of difference. Let's experiment with what happens when you listen to understand.

TRY THIS

Listening to Understand:
Building the Skill of Compassionate Listening

As you go about your day, be alert for opportunities to listen to others. You may find it easier to start with friends or others before you practice listening to your partner. As you build skill, remember to try it out with your partner too.

When you notice someone has something to say and you'd like to practice listening, see if you can remember your intention to listen to understand. This is a listening exercise, so resist the urge to speak.

Set an intention to listen to understand. Remember the

four Cs: centered, curious, connected, and compassionate. Remembering the four Cs and setting your intention may help you center yourself. Do you feel centered? If not, please place a hand on your heart, follow your breath, or feel your feet—whatever you need to center yourself.

As you turn your attention toward the speaker, notice what they look like. So much of communication is nonverbal. Do they look at ease, or is there tension in their face and body? What feeling state is their body communicating to you? A hot red face may mean embarrassment or anger; a tear in the eye may mean sadness or that they are deeply moved, for example. What do you notice about the state they are in?

If the speaker appears to be distressed and an urge arises in you to comfort or console them in some way, notice that is compassion arising in you. Let your heart open to this person without moving into comforting and soothing them right now.

Trust that your kind and caring presence is enough right now.

If you find that you are becoming distressed by what they are saying, see if you can stay with them and care for yourself by adding in a compassion practice. Try breathing in something you need—like courage or reassurance—with each inbreath. And then breathe out something you'd like to offer them—like relief of pain or love—with each outbreath. This could also be a color, a sensation of warmth, or a beautiful sunset. Anything you or they need. You can adjust the ratio as needed. You may just need to breathe in for yourself for a while as you listen to them. Or you may want to focus more on breathing out something good for them. See what feels right to you.

If you are still feeling overwhelmed by what they are saying, you may want to put a hand on your heart or offer yourself some kind and reassuring words. Or maybe it would feel best to feel your feet on the floor or tune in to the sensation of breathing. See what feels right for you. Stay as long as you can be with them while still in your window of tolerance. You can always stop listening if it becomes overwhelming and you aren't able to find a practice that helps you stay present *and* in your window of tolerance. Remember staying within your window of tolerance helps to build skill rather than wire in distress.

Remember that the intention is to learn more about the speaker. This isn't about you.

Now tune in to what the speaker is actually saying. Bring an attitude of curiosity to the act of listening and see if you can understand their perspective or experience.

Notice any thoughts that arise about what they are saying—especially arguments in your mind—and let those go. Remember that this is about understanding them rather than agreeing with them. Tune back in to what they are actually saying. You may need to do this again and again to better understand where they are coming from.

If you notice that scenarios from your own life are arising, that what they are saying is reminding you of similar times in your own life, that is common humanity arising. It's great that you can relate to what they are saying. It comes out of feeling connected. You're likely feeling a sense of "just like me." And it's also important to keep the focus on the speaker, so please resist the urge to share those scenarios right now.

Now see if you can broaden your attention even further. What do you know about this person? If it is someone you know well, you may understand this to be touching on a core pain in their life—something they've struggled with for a much of their life. Is there a reason that this event they are describing has a deeper meaning or impact for them? Can you take in the context of why this matters so much for them?

Watch for signs they are done speaking without stopping their process. They may pause to consider what they want to say next. It's good to give them space for that. You may find they go deeper and deeper into their experience when you do so. That's great, because you'll learn much more about them when they do. With practice you'll be able to pick up the cues that they are done speaking. They may look at you and say, "Thank

you." Or they may relax a bit. When they are done speaking—
and only when they are done speaking—it is your turn.

If you understood what they were saying, you can reflect
that back to them, validate them, or otherwise let them know
you've understood them and you care about them. For example, you might say something like "Wow, that sounds really
hard. I didn't realize how it felt for you. Thank you for trusting
me with that." Or whatever feels right to you. Remember this
still isn't about you.

If you don't have a sense of what they were saying or are
confused about something, now is your chance to ask clarifying
questions. You might say something like "I don't understand
what you were saying about _____, but I do want to
understand. Could you say more about _____?" or "Did
you mean _____?" Remember this is still about them,
and the questions are about clarifying your understanding of
them rather than a chance to rebut what they were saying.

When you've taken in what they are saying, the state they are
in, and the larger context, you may have a sense of what they
need right now. It's still good to check that out with them to be
sure what you want to offer them *is* what they need. You might
say something like "Is there anything you need right now?" or
you might be more specific and ask, "Would you like a hug?" As
best you can, offer whatever compassion feels right for both
of you.

There may still be lingering feelings on your end, and you may
need a chance to speak about what arose in you. If so, make
sure there is sufficient space between being the listener and
being the speaker. It's often best to wait until later in the day or
the following day to take your own turn at speaking.

Take a moment to notice any effects of this practice. How was
it different from how you ordinarily listen? Were there any benefits

for you in listening this way? Were there any benefits for the speaker? How might listening in this way impact your relationship?

Putting Speaking and Listening Together with Compassionate Communication

Now that you've had a chance to practice compassionate speaking and compassionate listening, it's a short step into compassionate communication. If you have a willing partner, you can practice compassionate communication with what my students have named "The 5-Minute Thing." That's because there is a kind of magic in practicing for 5 minutes. It's long enough to ride the wave of reactivity that may arise and refocus on what your partner is saying, but short enough that it feels doable to listen for 5 minutes.

If your partner isn't willing to practice these skills with you, that's okay too. You can practice with a friend if you like. Either way, know that your own practices of compassionate speaking and compassionate listening are bound to have an impact on your partner and the relationship. Both compassionate speaking and compassionate listening have the power to change a downward spiral into an upward spiral or avoid the downward spiral altogether. When we show up in an openhearted way—as the speaker or the listener—we become safer for our partners. And allowing ourselves to be seen in this way creates the foundation for intimacy to arise.

> Both compassionate speaking and compassionate listening can change a downward spiral into an upward one.

TRY THIS

The 5-Minute Thing—Compassionate Communication

You'll need to set aside 20 minutes with your partner for this exercise. You may want to schedule a time when you will have no distractions.

It's important to remember that this is a time to practice building the skills of compassionate communication—you aren't trying to solve a problem or otherwise come to a particular outcome. You're just practicing speaking and listening with compassion.

You may want to start with a few minutes of breathing, putting your hand on your heart or anywhere that feels supportive—as a reminder of your intention to pay kind and loving attention to yourself and your partner.

Decide who will be the speaker first and who will be the listener. The speaker takes a moment to prepare to speak. The speaker may want to go through the compassionate speaking exercise, STOP and LOVE, to prepare, or use what they wrote when they did the exercise earlier, if applicable.

When ready, if you're the speaker:

Take a moment to center yourself, then become curious about what is happening for you at a deeper level. Remind yourself that your partner is someone you love and are loved by, and set the intention to speak with an attitude of gentleness. Tend to what you would find compassionate, letting the listener know what you need.

If you are the listener:

Take a moment to center yourself, then become curious, becoming a detective trying to understand what the speaker is communicating. Foster connection by reminding yourself that the speaker is someone you love and are loved by even when distress arises. Remember that "just like me," this person is doing their best and is trying to find happiness and freedom from suffering. Then tend to your partner with compassion, considering what your partner needs.

The first 5 minutes:

The first 5 minutes are for the speaker to speak whatever is in their heart and mind and the listener to just listen. Please practice in the way you've learned to speak and listen with compassion. The speaker can take their time, speak when and how they like, pause when they need, and speak again.

The listener is just listening. Please resist the urge to speak or to touch your partner and let your partner have the fullness of their experience.

Set a timer for 5 minutes. Whenever the speaker feels ready, you can begin. When the timer goes off, take a moment to notice what it was like to speak in this way if you were the speaker or listen in this way if you were the listener. (No need to discuss this now. Just notice.)

The second 5 minutes:

The second 5 minutes are a chance for the listener to ask questions to better understand what the speaker is trying to communicate. The focus is still on the speaker rather than the listener's experience. If the listener understands the speaker and an urge arises to offer your partner comfort or reassurance (compassion), please check with the speaker first to be sure that is what they want, then feel free to offer them compassion.

Remember to set the timer for 5 minutes. When the timer goes off, let that be enough for now. Pause and notice what happened for you in this section. Then take a few nice, easy breaths, letting go of the situation you just discussed and finding your way back into this moment and this body.

The third 5 minutes:

Now you'll switch roles. The speaker becomes the listener and the listener becomes the speaker. You can prepare yourself for your new role by taking a few minutes to tune in to your breath or by putting a hand on your body.

The speaker chooses what to talk about. This can be something completely different than what the partner just shared. That's often skillful. The speaker can use the STOP and LOVE practice to prepare to speak or use what they wrote in the compassionate speaking exercise.

These next 5 minutes are for the speaker to speak

whatever is in their heart and mind and the listener to just listen. Please practice in the way you've learned to speak and listen with compassion. The speaker can take their time, speak when and how they like, pause when they need, and speak again.

The listener is just listening. Please resist the urge to speak or to touch your partner and let them have the fullness of their experience.

Set a timer for 5 minutes. Whenever the speaker feels ready, you can begin. When the timer goes off, take a moment to notice what it was like to speak in this way if you were the speaker. Or listen in this way if you were the listener. (No need to discuss this now. Just notice.)

The fourth 5 minutes:

These last 5 minutes are a chance for the listener to ask questions to better understand what the speaker is trying to communicate. The focus is still on the speaker rather than the listener's experience. If the listener understands the speaker and an urge arises to offer your partner comfort or reassurance (compassion), please check with the speaker first to be sure that is what they want—then feel free to offer them compassion.

Remember to set the timer for 5 minutes. When the timer goes off, let that be enough for now. Pause and notice what happened for you in this section. Then take a few nice, easy breaths, letting go of the situation you just discussed and finding your way back into this moment and this body.

At the end of this exercise, most couples want to take some time to discuss what they experienced in this practice. If the urge arises to delve into what was shared and work it through to an outcome, please resist the urge. Doing so will interfere with the process the next time you set aside time to practice compassionate communication. Instead, you may find it helpful to talk about your experiences of speaking and listening in this 5-minute format. Share what worked for you and what didn't.

Then, if needed, customize the practice to your own needs as you move forward.

Remember to start small. Start with the less threatening conversations, whether that be with your partner or a friend. As you experience success you'll gradually build confidence and skill and will be ready to gradually work your way into discussing more difficult topics. It's best to build from success rather than rush the process and have a negative outcome. It takes practice, and frequency is more important than difficulty when building the new habit of communicating with compassion.

Barbara Fredrickson has said, "Once two people understand each other—really 'get' each other in any given moment—the benevolent concerns and actions of mutual care can flow forth unimpeded." That's been my experience too.

When we use a technique to get a certain outcome, our partners may come away feeling like a subtle (or not so subtle) attempt at manipulation is happening. When instead we focus on the process of opening our hearts to each other—seeing the other person, understanding them, and meeting them with love—we are much more likely to "get" each other. When we feel safely connected—seen, understood, accepted, and loved—we naturally want to connect with our partner and tend to our shared well-being.

In my work with couples, I've been amazed at how even the most poorly worded attempt at speaking up has been met with kindness, understanding, and compassion when the listener can feel the underlying intention of love and care from the speaker (and how even the most beautifully worded attempt has flopped spectacularly when the listener can feel the underlying feelings of blame or resentment).

Please hold all of these exercises lightly. They are designed to help you find that openhearted place. In the end you'll need to let go of technique and find what helps you hold yourself, your partner, and your relationship with love or get back to that place when you've gotten off course. When you do, it really changes everything. At the heart of things, we all just want to be loved and accepted.

11

"Can We Heal Our Wounds?"

Cultivating the Conditions
for Forgiveness

Forgiving is not forgetting; it's actually remembering—
remembering and not using your right to hit back. It's a
second chance for a new beginning. And the remembering
part is particularly important. Especially if you don't want
to repeat what happened.

—Archbishop Desmond Tutu

Imagine if you still had an open wound from every scratch, scrape, or
cut you've endured in your lifetime. Your physical body would likely
be a mess. And there is a good chance the cumulative pain would be
nearly unbearable. It's important that the body have a mechanism for
healing. After all, no one gets through life without some scratches and
scrapes, and some of us have it much worse than that.

In a similar way we don't get through life without emotional
wounds. Relationships are breeding grounds for emotional wounds
and also can provide the support for emotional healing. Our primary
relationships are especially fertile ground for experiencing injuries.
The more important someone is to us, the more vulnerable we are to
being hurt by them. In spite of our good intentions and our growing
skills, we will sometimes injure each other. It is important to have
skills in repairing our relationships when inevitable injuries arise.

Remember, we are imperfect beings who are wired to fight,

flee, or freeze when we feel unsafe. We are capable of such harmful actions—saying critical things that wound our partners to the core, withdrawing our affection, and freezing our partners out. Or worse, turning our affection to someone else, betraying that sacred promise we made. The list of potential ways to wound or be wounded in a relationship is seemingly endless.

And yet most often there is also good in the relationship. Shared histories or families, those qualities that drew you to your partner originally—your partner's sense of humor, kindness, courage, or reliability, whatever it may be for you. Often there is enough good left that we stay in the relationship. However, when we don't know how to repair the hurts, we carry an ever-growing bundle of injuries with us. Unable to heal and unable to leave, we can feel stuck in purgatory. Feeling ever more unsafe in the relationship, we maintain a certain distance, and maintaining a certain distance we feel a deep sense of loneliness and disconnection. Often we carry anger and resentment as a way to help us remember to maintain that distance.

The Buddha is quoted as having said, "Holding on to anger is like grasping a hot coal with the intent of throwing it at someone else; you are the one who gets burned." He also reportedly said, "Holding on to anger is like drinking poison and expecting the other person to die." The point is that holding on to chronic anger and resentment is harmful to us. Beyond the emotional and relational consequences of chronic anger and resentment, the body isn't meant to be constantly dosed with stress hormones, which are known to cause health issues. Far from keeping us safe, our resentment harms us.

Forgiveness is the salve that can heal those wounds and repair the relationship. I don't say that lightly. Perhaps, like me, you were taught to "forgive and forget." How'd that work out for you? I hated it. To me it translated as an instruction to push down the pain I'd endured and slap on a happy face. Pushing down the pain doesn't heal anything. The wound just festers in the dark. So that isn't the kind of forgiveness I'm talking about here. In fact quite the opposite; the wound needs tending to or it just won't heal.

If you've been following along in this book, you have been building a skill base that will help you deal with the injuries in a way that feels safer. Safety is important! No one wants to be injured again, especially in the same way. Tolerating harm doesn't benefit anyone. We'll build on that skill base and explore how to engage safely with forgiveness practices. But first, let's look at why you may not want to forgive.

Misgivings about Forgiveness

Most of us have blocks to forgiveness. When invited to engage in the process of forgiveness we can feel a certain resistance. It's important to understand and address our blocks. Please take a moment to identify what underlies resistance to forgiving for you. Here are some common blocks:

Justice: "It would be unjust to forgive; I don't want to let that person get away with it."

Forgiveness doesn't let people off the hook for the harm they've caused. It doesn't subvert or preclude justice. It opens space for a process of justice that is uncorrupted by the press for vengeance.

Weakness: "Forgiving is weak."

Facing the injury we have suffered and the pain that goes with it actually requires a great deal of strength and courage.

Condoning: "Forgiving would mean saying what happened is okay."

True forgiveness does not condone or excuse bad behavior. It recognizes the humanity of the person who engaged in the behavior. It says, "You are okay, even if your behavior is not okay."

Withholding: "They hurt me. I'm not interested in giving them anything."

Although forgiveness is a gift, we need not focus on what it offers the other person. In fact, as in the case of forgiving one who has passed away, forgiveness can occur with no involvement from the one who injured us. We can choose to forgive solely because of an awareness of the ways we ourselves suffer when our hearts are constricted, defended, resentful, and unforgiving. Forgiveness is the path to freedom.

Protection: "If I forgive him, it will happen again."

Forgiveness does not mean letting go of needed boundaries and putting yourself in an unsafe situation. It also does not mean we must stay in a relationship with the person who has injured us. It isn't the same as reconciliation. The final step in the forgiveness process is to renew or release the relationship, and we must decide for ourselves what is wisest.

Forgetting: "I can never forget the harm she caused me."

Forgiveness isn't the same as forgetting. In fact, when we are freed from the anger and resentment, it can become possible to transform the deep pain of experiencing harm into love and meaning. From this place we can also help others heal. In fact, remembering is important because it can help us help others. My friend and colleague Margaret Cullen, developer of the Mindfulness-Based Emotional Balance program, notes, "Forgiveness is not forgetting. Forgiveness is how you hold in your heart something that is wrong while you take the necessary steps to correct it and to help prevent it from happening again."

Inability: "I can't forgive. I've tried, and I don't have it in me."

Everyone has the capacity to forgive. We can't will forgiveness, but we can be willing to forgive. Forgiveness takes time. Often we must move through several cycles of remembering, grief, and unforgiveness before we are free.

Forgiveness is a process. Trying to force yourself to forgive your partner or your partner to forgive you will just bring added pain. You have a responsibility to tend to your safety, and if you feel forgiveness itself will make you unsafe, it will be nearly impossible to forgive.

In fact, true forgiveness can make you safer. You still need to tend to your own safety through good boundaries and other means. As I've said earlier in this book, safety is a precondition for compassion. Forgiveness is not a substitute for safety. Please do whatever you need to tend to your own physical and emotional safety. Forgiveness can offer you safety from the inner prison of anger and resentment.

Cultivating the Conditions for Forgiveness

You can't will yourself to forgive (or your partner to forgive you!). And anger and resentment don't have an expiration date. Until the wound has been tended, the injury is still alive in the present for us, no matter how long ago it happened. The best we can do is to cultivate the conditions for forgiveness and open to our willingness to forgive. Then it happens in its own time. As Margaret Cullen pointed out when I interviewed her for the Well Connected Relationships podcast, it's normal to feel forgiveness one moment and slide back into a state of unforgiveness the next. Gradually through engaging in the process of forgiveness, we spend more time in forgiveness than nonforgiveness. This can take a lifetime, and some wounds are so large that we don't arrive in forgiveness at all. Still this process of softening the heart and tending to the wound can alleviate our suffering.

It's a process that requires tending. Much like the garden requires regular watering for the seeds to grow, cultivating forgiveness requires tending to the conditions of forgiveness.

It probably comes as no surprise by now that I like to look at things through the lens of mindfulness, common humanity, and kindness. Let's take a look at forgiveness through that lens now.

Mindfulness

While many of us are motivated to forgive in hopes that we can get out of pain, we can't actually skip over the pain. If we are to heal, we must open to the injury itself. There is a saying, "What we feel we can heal." This is true in our relationships, too. When we open to feeling our own pain and our partner's pain, we open the door to healing. That very presence with our pain and that of our partner is the first step to cultivating the conditions of forgiveness.

So often, however, we don't want to see the pain. We don't want to know that we have caused harm. When we open to our partner's pain, we may feel the pain of empathic resonance. It is actually painful to feel the pain of someone we love. It's especially painful if we were the cause of the pain. Avoiding our partner's pain is often an attempt to avoid the shame of knowing we caused our loved one harm. Or maybe it is our own pain we are avoiding, rather than our partner's pain. Often there is a sense of hopelessness underneath that avoidance. We don't believe that being vulnerable and opening to the pain will actually result in healing.

"What's the use?" we ask ourselves as we prepare our stiff upper lip and move on.

Avoiding seeing our partners' pain is a way of avoiding the shame of having caused that pain.

On the other end of things, we may be quick to admit fault and quick to try to fix it. We may even offer an apology. Have you ever found yourself using this strategy? Have you ever been on the receiving end of this strategy? How did it feel? Unless our partners open to and acknowledge our pain and the damage caused by their behavior, their apologies can feel like a strategy to avoid taking responsibility. Like using the "get out of jail free" card in the game of Monopoly, our partners may wish to avoid dealing with the consequences of their actions and go straight to "forgive and forget." This is the opposite of presence (mindfulness).

Working Mindfully with Our Own Injury

What we need when we are injured is to have our injury acknowledged. We need to know our partners care about us and care about our well-being. We don't want to be left to hold our pain alone. Their presence with our pain can foster the beginning of the return of safety for us. If we are not sure that our partners will care and hold the pain with us, it is much harder to be vulnerable with them. This can really erode intimacy.

It can be challenging to talk about how we've been hurt. When we have been hurt, and especially when we don't feel safe being vulnerable, we tend to speak from the threat/defense system. Fight, flight, and freeze is in play. We may attack with our words, avoid the subject of our pain altogether, or placate in an effort to avoid conflict. Instead it is helpful to speak, but in a way that doesn't activate defensiveness in our partner. The compassionate speaking introduced in Chapter 10 can be really helpful here.

When we are the injured party, we need to speak from a place of vulnerability. Often we focus on our partners' behavior and how they messed up because it makes us feel less vulnerable than revealing how much pain we are in. However, our anger is likely to push them away . . . like the porcupine with its quills out. It is much easier to approach someone who is injured than someone who is blaming.

Finding safety through tending to our own needs is important. We may choose to practice self-compassion before speaking with our partners about the injury and what we need. This can give us the emotional resources to tolerate the vulnerable position of revealing our pain to our partners. Speaking from the vulnerable place of how we are injured requires great courage. When we can come from this place, we have a much greater chance of being heard and having our injury acknowledged.

Working Mindfully with Our Partners' Injury

As challenging as it can be to speak up, it is often much more painful to listen to the pain we have caused our partners. It is common to want to protect our ego from shame and guilt, which often activates the fight/flight/freeze system in the listener. Also, to protect ourselves from feeling their pain, it can be tempting to go into fixing. If we can make their pain go away, then we don't have to feel it anymore. What our partners really need is for us to listen in a way that truly receives them.

When our partners reveal their pain to us, it is an intimate act. They are giving us the gift of letting us come closer to them. We need to be sure we honor that gift by responding in a caring way. Doing so may require some work on our part.

The best way to care for our partners is to offer our presence. If we can set aside our own ego and make the other person more important than our self-image, we can become curious about that person and their pain. The compassionate listening exercise in Chapter 10 can be really helpful here.

It isn't always comfortable to hear about our partners' pain, especially when we caused it. It takes courage to be with pain we may have caused for as long as they need us to hear them. We can listen, and when they are done speaking—really done speaking—we can let them know we see and hear their pain. We can show we care about them. We can own anything we need to take responsibility for in terms of mistakes we have made, and we can let them know we understand the pain that our behavior has caused them.

> Opening to your partner's pain makes you less likely to repeat the mistake you made, which makes your partner feel safer and creates a foundation for repair.

This is an important step. We are much less likely to repeat the mistake if we fully open to the pain it causes our partners. Therefore, opening to the fullness of our partners' pain increases the likelihood that they will be safe in the relationship. Listening is truly an act of love. So mindfully opening to the injury sets the foundation for repair.

Common Humanity

When we have been harmed, it is tempting to think of ourselves as victims and our partners as perpetrators. Of course, in any given situation sometimes one person was the victim and the other the perpetrator. However, victim or perpetrator isn't really who any of us are. We aren't only injured or only harmful. No matter how kindhearted and well-intentioned we are, no one gets through life without having injured others as well as being injured. As humans we end up both injuring and being injured, and when we fall into the victim identity we don't see, claim, or understand our own capacity to cause harm and feel regret. Similarly, when we see the harm we have caused and are consumed by guilt and shame, we aren't able to hold our good qualities along with our undesirable actions. This sense of separateness only adds to the pain and blocks the opportunity for repair.

When we can acknowledge that the shared human condition includes having both strengths and shortcomings, it is easier to feel compassion for ourselves and others. Rather than putting your partner or yourself in the "bad" category, the task is to see everyone in the context of our humanness, with strengths and shortcomings. That doesn't mean we gloss over the injury—we do need to open to it mindfully. But when we do, we can make a distinction between the harmful behavior and the person who caused the harm.

The Common Humanity of Making Mistakes

In any given moment when our suffering exceeds our resources, unskillful behavior (which we sometimes call "bad behavior") is likely to be the result. This is part of the human condition. What we are capable of on a day when everything is going well for us is not the same as what we are capable of on a day when everything is going wrong. So one thing to consider is the current conditions in the life of those who cause us injury. Were they in the midst of a stressful time in life and not as skillful as they might otherwise be?

At the same time, we are also impacted by our history. We are more tender in certain places when we have had similar injuries in the past. Our tenderness isn't our fault. No one asks to be injured in relationships. We had the childhood we had. We have the history we have. We are doing our best to work with that, and when we know better we can do better. Paul Gilbert, referred to throughout Part I of this book, speaks to this when he writes that had he been born into different circumstances he too may have become a gang member capable of killing others. Not everyone has been given the same opportunities in life. Not everyone has had the chance to feel safe in relationships. So another thing to consider is the personal history of the person who caused the injury. Were there external forces that shaped this person's personality?

Beyond our personal history, there is our family and cultural history. Through our connections with them, the pain and unskillful ways of being are passed on, often through generations. It is also skillful to consider the larger context of life for the person who caused the injury (you or your partner). We must see how we also behave in unskillful ways and how, given the right current and historical conditions, we could have caused this injury. Doing so softens the heart a bit with understanding.

Remember, we aren't saying that the injury or the behavior that caused the injury was okay. We can and should take steps to prevent that injury from happening again. Rather, we are noticing that the human who caused the injury wasn't acting alone; instead the person is part of a larger system, which has also influenced how skillful that person could be at the time.

The Common Humanity of Feeling Hurt

Being hurt is also part of common humanity. We are wired to feel pain when we are abandoned or criticized, for example. These things are threats to our well-being and threats to our relationships. When we feel hurt by these things, it doesn't mean something is wrong with us. It means that we are fully human and things are working the way they should.

Some people carry much more hurt about a given situation than others, and we need to stay out of judgment about whether the degree of hurt is justified. How hurt we are also depends on the current conditions of our life. When things are going well for us, it tends to be easier to take difficulties in stride. When things are not going well, sometimes every little injury feels huge.

Here too we are impacted by our history. When we have been injured in a relationship, especially in similar ways, we can become fine-tuned to pick up on even the slightest infraction. These injuries are also passed down by our parents and our culture. For example, a girl whose mother has been injured by men is often told not to let men take advantage of her. In this way the injury is passed down from mother to daughter. These passed-down lessons can be lifesaving. They can also heighten our anxiety about being injured and instill a sense of mistrust in us.

It is important that those who are injured be met with generosity and understanding. If you consider their history along with their current conditions, it makes sense that they are injured. We must also see how we would likely feel the same injury, had we been subject to the same conditions.

Kindness

When we open to the injury and we hold our partners and ourselves in the context of common humanity, a warmth of understanding often arises and we feel the urge to help. Where before the urge to take action came out of a place of avoiding pain, now the urge to take action comes out of embracing the pain and, more importantly, the person who is in pain.

It is important that we be in our care system before trying to engage in mending things with another person. Therefore, it is often helpful to pause and tend to ourselves with self-compassion before proceeding to tend to repair of the injury.

Taking Action to Mend and Repair

As we move into the action part of kindness we consider what is needed here and what would be skillful. At the same time, we are no longer attached to the outcome. Now we are landing in loving, connected presence. Our very kind presence alone is an act of love and generosity. And sometimes that presence is all that is needed. Other times the repair requires taking responsibility for our actions by apologizing.

Apologizing Skillfully

Apologizing doesn't mean taking a one-down position or considering yourself a horrible human being. On the contrary, that would make your apology all about you. Apologizing is a natural outcome of tending to the needs of the injured party. A good apology:

- Takes responsibility for the action that caused the harm without excusing those actions
- Acknowledges the harm that your actions have caused your partner in a way that validates your partner's feelings and the resulting injuries
- Takes responsibility for taking actions that will prevent the harm from recurring, thereby tending to the safety of the person who was harmed
- Seeks to understand and honor what your partner needs now
- Allows your partner the time and space necessary to heal

Forgiving Skillfully

Being able to forgive frees us from the burden of carrying anger and resentment. It also creates a new foundation for renewal of the relationship—should that be what you decide is in your best interest. It's hard to get closer to someone when you are filled with anger and resentment.

It's important to remember that forgiveness is a process rather than a destination. We can't *make* ourselves or each other forgive. And we don't need to forget or allow ourselves to be harmed again. We have a responsibility to attend to our own safety and to prevent and alleviate our own harm, as much as possible.

> Forgiveness is a process, not a destination, and the process cannot be forced.

You can ask yourself whether you feel ready to begin the forgiveness process. Forgiveness should not be approached from a place of "having to" forgive. Forgiveness comes from the heart, so it requires an openness to wanting to be able to forgive. If you don't have the desire to begin the process, that's okay. Just know that carrying the burden of anger and resentment will get in the way of being able to get close to your partner again.

It may be that what you need at this point is to focus on reestablishing safety for yourself and in your relationship. Forgiveness is not a substitute for safety. When you do feel ready to begin the process, the following steps can be helpful:

1. Start by attending to your own safety. Know that you will not allow yourself to be harmed again to the best of your ability.
2. From that place of safety, open mindfully to the pain you are in and offer yourself compassion.
3. Aware of the cost to you of continuing to carry the pain and resentment, set an intention to let go of this burden.
4. Consider the causes and conditions that might be underneath your partner's harmful behavior.
5. Open slowly to beginning to offer forgiveness.

Remember that it is a process and that it is normal to toggle back and forth between forgiving and being unwilling to forgive. As best you can, accept yourself just as you are, whatever state you are in. One poem that speaks to the challenge of being willing to forgive is this beautiful work by Desmond and Mpho Tutu in *The Book of Forgiving:*

Prayer Before the Prayer

I want to be willing to forgive
But I dare not ask for the will to forgive
In case you give it to me
And I am not yet ready
I am not yet ready for my heart to soften
I am not yet ready to be vulnerable again
Not yet ready to see that there is humanity in my tormentor's eyes
Or that the one who hurt me may also have cried
I am not yet ready for the journey
I am not yet interested in the path
I am at the prayer before the prayer of forgiveness
Grant me the will to want to forgive
Grant it to me not yet but soon
Can I even form the words?
Forgive me?
Dare I even look?
Do I dare to see the hurt I have caused?
I can glimpse all the shattered pieces of that fragile thing
That soul trying to rise on the broken wings of hope
But only out of the corner of my eye
I am afraid of it
And if I am afraid to see
How can I not be afraid to say
Forgive me?

Is there a place where we can meet?
You and me
The place in the middle
The no man's land
Where we straddle the lines
Where you are right
And I am right too.
And both of us are wrong and wronged
Can we meet there?

And look for the place where the path begins
The path that ends when we forgive

Putting Forgiveness into Practice

When you do feel ready to open to the process of forgiving your partner or forgiving yourself, it's important to work with the smaller injuries first. As we build skills and resources we can move toward the bigger injuries; however, it's best to start with the easier end of the spectrum.

Before opening to the practice, it is skillful to consider whether you have the emotional resources to begin this exercise right now. If not, please give yourself what you need right now. You can always come back and do this exercise later, when you are feeling more resourced.

If you feel ready, let's begin with a practice to help you forgive others.

TRY THIS
Forgiving Others

Audio Track 23

Begin by finding a comfortable position and settling in whichever way feels best to you. You might choose to follow your breath for a bit, to feel the sensations where your body makes contact with whatever is holding you up, or perhaps you would like to open to sounds in the room. Choose whichever practice best helps you center yourself and open to the present moment.

When you are ready, call to mind something small to medium that your partner has done that hurt you. Please don't make this something traumatic. Let's stay on the easier end of the spectrum here. This could also mean working with someone else who has hurt you and working with a specific event.

Please be sure to choose something you would like to forgive, if possible.

Contact the pain that this person has caused you, perhaps feeling it in your body as residual stress.

If it feels right, offer yourself a kind and supportive touch, perhaps placing your hand on the part of the body that is holding the stress and allowing kindness to flow from your hand to your body. Feel the support of the touch.

Begin offering yourself compassion for how you've suffered, perhaps saying, "May I be safe, may I be peaceful, may I be kind to myself, may I accept myself as I am" or using your own phrases.

If it feels like you need to stay here, keep giving yourself compassion for as long as you need.

If it still feels right, begin to forgive by considering the burden to you as you carry the hurt and resentment of the injury. If it is helpful and you feel ready to let go of that burden, perhaps say something to yourself like "I've carried this pain long enough. I'm ready to set it down now."

See if you can see the other person more clearly and understand the forces that led this person to act in a way that hurt you badly. Recognize it is human to make mistakes.

What were the current conditions in this person's life? For example, were they under a lot of stress at the time?

What were the factors that may have shaped this person's personality? For example, did this person have a difficult childhood?

Were there any cultural or societal factors that shaped this person, like being marginalized or oppressed?

If your heart begins to soften with the understanding that we all make mistakes when our suffering exceeds our resources, know that the other person's mistake—while not acceptable—was a human mistake.

If it feels right, begin to offer forgiveness to the other person, perhaps saying the phrase "May I begin to forgive you for what you have done that has caused me harm." Or it might feel better to say, "May I begin to open to the possibility of forgiving you for what you have done that has caused me harm." Or you could say, "I offer you forgiveness to the extent that I am ready." See what feels right to you.

When you feel ready, take a few moments to rest here by

going back to following the breath, feeling yourself grounded and safely held by the chair or cushion you are sitting on or offering yourself your own kind touch or words.

Know that you can and will tend to your own safety, as best you can, moving forward. Consider what that means for you in this relationship right now.

You may want to take a moment and pause here to take any notes that would be helpful. Please remember that this is a process and don't worry about the outcome. When we practice forgiveness, we are training the heart to put down the burden we are carrying. If you did feel unburdened by this practice, please make a note of how releasing the resentment you are carrying has freed you in some way.

While it can be helpful to work toward forgiving your partner, sometimes the person you need to forgive is yourself. It's also difficult to get close to your partner when you are carrying guilt or shame about how your actions caused your partner harm. Sometimes we get so wrapped in our own guilt and shame—and our defenses against opening to and feeling our regret and remorse—that we can't really see the other person anymore. So we end up carrying the burden of shame, our partner ends up all alone with the hurt, and the relationship grows more distant. Forgiving yourself can help you heal so that you can help your partner heal and also rebuild and repair the relationship. If you feel ready, let's try that now.

TRY THIS
Forgiving Yourself

Audio Track 24

Begin by taking a moment to ground yourself and come into the present moment in whatever way works best for you. You can return to feeling your body breathing, placing a hand on your heart or elsewhere, feeling yourself supported by the cushion or chair, or opening to sounds, for example. Spend a few minutes coming into the present moment and centering and grounding yourself.

When you are ready, call to mind something for which you would like to forgive yourself. For instance, you might be feeling some remorse about what happened with the person you practiced with in the Forgiving Others exercise. Perhaps that person didn't bring out the best in you and you know it. If you feel no guilt or responsibility for what happened, please focus on another situation in which you feel some remorse for how you behaved. Again it is best to practice with something mild to moderate to begin with.

Take a few moments to consider how your actions impacted the other person and allow yourself to feel your regret and remorse.

While opening to the truth of what you did, also recognize that it's human to make mistakes. Maybe you feel some shame. That's also human. Notice the burden you are carrying.

Begin to offer yourself compassion for how you have suffered, perhaps saying, "May I be free from fear, may I be free from shame, may I be kind to myself, may I accept myself as I am," or whatever feels right to you here.

If it feels like you need to stay here, keep giving yourself compassion.

When you are ready, try to see yourself more clearly and understand some factors leading to your mistake. Take a moment to consider:

Were there any current factors causing you to be less skillful than usual—for example, were you under a lot of stress?

Were certain aspects of your personality triggered in an irrational way? Were old buttons pushed?

Were there any cultural or societal factors that impacted your capacity, like a history of being marginalized or oppressed in some way?

If your heart begins to soften with the understanding that we all make mistakes when our suffering exceeds our resources, know that your mistake—while not acceptable—was a human mistake.

Now see if you can offer forgiveness to yourself, saying the phrase "May I begin to forgive myself for what I have done that caused this person harm." Or maybe you need to start with "May I begin to open to the possibility of forgiving myself."

When you feel ready, take a few moments to rest here by going back to following the breath, feeling yourself grounded and safely held by the chair or cushion you are sitting on or offering yourself your own kind touch.

Know that you can and will tend to keeping this person and yourself safe, as best you can, moving forward. Consider what that means for you in this relationship right now.

You may want to take a moment and pause here to take any notes that would be helpful. Please remember that this is a process and don't worry about the outcome. When we practice forgiveness, we are training the heart to put down the burden we are carrying. If you did feel unburdened by this practice, please make a note of how releasing the guilt and shame you may be carrying has freed you in some way. Notice if it has made it possible for you to open more fully to the pain your partner is carrying and if it makes it possible for you to move back in toward the relationship, rather than keeping yourself removed in some way.

The Power of Forgiveness and Repair

While forgiveness and repair are a process that unfolds in its own time, we do have some influence in how long and whether or not that repair happens. Please don't despair if it doesn't happen right away. Each time you practice, you water the seeds of forgiveness. Over time the soil becomes softer and more fertile. The key is to let go of the outcome and practice because you, your partner, and your relationship matter to you. The seeds will blossom when they blossom. Keep practicing, because the benefits are tremendous. There is a path to reconciliation and repair. There is a path back to intimacy.

12

"How Do We Keep Our Love Alive?"

Celebrating Positive Experiences Together

> Let us be grateful to the people who make us happy; they are the charming gardeners who make our souls blossom.
> —MARCEL PROUST

I'd been seeing Chelle and Sergio in couples therapy for a few months now. It had been a bumpy ride. It was clear that they'd fallen madly in love with each other, and then when the stress of life hit, things didn't go so well. Sergio was a house painter. He worked hard, but with a fairly predictable schedule, and he enjoyed his work. By nature he was calm and reliable. This was one of the things that attracted Chelle to him. Chelle had more ambition and with it more anxiety. She was in the corporate world and worked hard. Sergio was proud of his wife and how strong and ambitious she was.

In the beginning her work was exciting, but in the last couple of years things had become really stressful at work. Actually, they had become overwhelming, and Chelle was really struggling to cope. At first she started having a glass of wine when she got home from work, but that turned out to be a slippery slope. The more her life fell apart the more she drank. And the more she drank the more her life fell apart. She'd had more than a few out-of-control incidents where she said and did things that were not only embarrassing but dangerous. Sergio was really concerned about his wife, especially when she didn't come home and she didn't call—which was becoming a regular event. He was terrified that she was in trouble, and he didn't know how to protect her. He'd tried letting her know how worried he was and even tried to talk with her about her drinking. She was the best thing that ever happened to him, and now he was losing her. He was worried that she wouldn't survive much longer.

Her individual therapist had referred them to me for couples therapy, and shortly after we began working together this whole thing unraveled. To their credit, they'd been facing these issues in our work together. It wasn't easy or smooth, but they showed up week after week and faced the pain in themselves, each other, and their relationship. We'd worked on many of the things we've already explored in this book, and things were improving greatly. Chelle was now in recovery and really working hard. They understood, accepted, and reassured each other now. They'd become much more skillful with each other, but there was still an air of dissatisfaction that hung in the air when they were together.

And then something remarkable happened. It was toward the end of one of our sessions, and almost as a throwaway comment Chelle explained that she had a week off work and that they really wanted to use that time to work on their marriage. She wondered if there was some sort of retreat or deep intensive work they could spend the week doing. I was struck by the intensity of their (her) drive to improve. It actually broke my heart a bit that when some space opened up for them they wanted to fill it with *more* hard work. They'd been working extremely hard for quite some time. What they really needed was a break. They needed some space to get back to the joy and connection they'd experienced earlier in their relationship.

I pushed back on the idea of more work. I told them they'd already been working really hard and they'd learned a lot and had come a long way. Could they allow themselves some space to rest, renew, connect, and enjoy each other's company? I wondered. They were shocked. I told them what I thought they really needed was to actually take the week off and go on vacation together. They looked a bit stunned but promised to consider it.

In the end they trusted me and went on vacation. The degree of healing that came from that one week of vacation surprised us all. In that week they reclaimed their well-being for themselves, each other, and their relationship. They opened again to the fullness of life. They opened again to the joy in life. They'd been focusing on the very real problems in their relationship and working really hard on them. And that was important. But that was all they could see. When they went on vacation together, their world expanded again and they could hold all of that struggle in the context of the deep love they had for each other. And they reclaimed their capacity to relax, connect, and play together.

Our work ended shortly after that vacation. They had what they needed. In the months and years that followed they were happy together. They bought a home, started a family, and settled into their new roles surrounded by love and gratitude. Something about having almost lost each other made their connection even sweeter. They were grateful.

Finding the Care System

In Part I of this book we spent a lot of time unpacking the emotion regulation systems: threat/defense, drive, and care. We looked at how we, our partners, and our relationships can get stuck in the threat/defense system. We also looked at how we often resist the pain of that system by enlisting the drive system to fix and control things in order to prevent or get out of pain. We looked at how, instead of resisting that very pain, it is important to open to it. And we explored how to use the care system to hold ourselves and our partners when pain is present. These ways of meeting pain with kindness (the very definition of compassion) can help us and our partners move from the threat/defense system to the care system with its characteristic feelings of safeness, contentment, and connectedness. When we use these techniques, over time, our relationships themselves can move from a baseline of the threat/defense system to the care system. This is what happened for Chelle and Sergio. The relationship itself, once stuck in the threat/defense system, moved into the care system when they rediscovered their capacity for connection through rest, renewal, and play. Coupled with the skills to tend to themselves and each other when pain arose, this rekindled capacity for shared joy and well-being tipped the scales into a relationship based in the care system.

Cultivating the "Magic Ratio"

Couples researcher John Gottman talks about the magic ratio of 5:1 in which secure and happy relationships are characterized by at least five positive interactions for every one negative interaction. The thing is that once the initial hormone cocktail of a new relationship wears off and we can see faults in our partners or our relationships, we can become so narrowly focused on these problems that we can no longer see or appreciate the positive qualities in our partners or our relationships. Getting stuck in this negativity bias is no fun. We do need to open to problems, in the way we have in this book. Problems are opportunities for growth and deepening intimacy. However, we need to create a base of positive interactions too. Especially if you've been stuck in a negative relational pattern with your partner, this involves *intentionally* cultivating and anchoring positive experiences. In this chapter we'll take a closer look at how to cultivate these positive interactions.

> We need to create a base of positive interactions, intentionally cultivating and anchoring positive experiences.

Mindfulness and Savoring

One aspect of mindfulness is awareness. When positive things happen in our lives, we tend to become accustomed to them and forget to notice them. This is the way we are wired. We often appreciate novel experiences because we're dosed with dopamine. But over time, we take them for granted and then fail to notice. For example, maybe your partner hates to do the dishes. You find yourself cooking the dinner and doing the dishes, and you're feeling burdened by "always" being the one to do the dishes. Then one night, without you asking, your partner gets up after the meal, clears the table, and does the dishes. Once you get over your surprise, you're likely to feel grateful. But if he takes on this new role and routinely does the dishes after dinner, at some point you're likely to take it for granted. And over time, you probably won't even notice him standing at the sink doing the dishes. It's lost its novelty.

Mindful Awareness

The point is that positive things are likely already happening in our lives and in our relationships and we are failing to notice them. Renowned mindfulness teacher Thich Nhat Hanh put it this way: "When we have a bad toothache, happiness is freedom from toothache. When we have freedom from toothache, we forget to be happy." So the first step is actually to notice when we have "freedom from toothache" or when our partners do the dishes.

However, mindfulness is much more than just simple awareness or noticing. Mindfulness is all about experiencing things as they are happening. It's the difference between knowing you are taking a shower and experiencing the shower by feeling the warmth of the water, the lather of the shampoo, and the slipperiness of the soap. When we are mindful, we are opening ourselves up to whatever experience we are having.

Mindfulness is the process of diving beneath our habits of numbing and avoiding so that we can feel and experience our lives. Without it our positive experiences often just flow down the drain.

Savoring

What happens when you do notice something like a beautiful sunset? Do you say to yourself, "Oh, beautiful sunset" and then keep walking by? Or do you allow yourself to stop and take in the positive experience, perhaps stopping and noticing the shape of the clouds and the colors of the horizon? This is called *savoring*, and it can make a big difference in our lives. Psychologist Rick Hanson refers to this as "taking in the good," and he notes that it takes as little as 30 seconds of

staying with a positive experience and
allowing ourselves to soak it in. When
we do this, we actually change our
implicit memory and begin to correct for
our negativity bias. When we savor positive experiences with our partners, we
come to experience the relationship as
more positive overall.

> Savoring positive
> experiences together,
> we come to experience
> the relationship as more
> positive in general.

Mindfulness and Savoring Practices

In the next practice we set a timer and allow ourselves to open to and
savor positive experiences as they arise for us. It's important to note
that we are not requiring ourselves to be positive or to find things we
like; rather we are simply opening to the possibilities and savoring
them when they come.

TRY THIS
Sense and Savor Walk

Start by finding a place, preferably in nature, where you feel
comfortable and at ease and are drawn to the setting. This
could be in a forest, or it could just as easily be in your back-
yard or at a neighborhood park. If weather or fatigue is an
issue, it could also be indoors at your kitchen table or resting
in your bedroom.

When you've arrived at that place, set a timer for a fixed
amount of time. This can be 5–15 minutes, depending on how
much time you have and your own comfort level. Longer times
allow us to open more fully to positive experiences.

Open your awareness to things around you, and as you do,
see where your attention naturally goes. If you're in your home,
it could be the feel of a warm blanket or the smell and taste of a
cup of tea. If you're in nature, it could be as open as the clouds
in the sky or as narrow as a dewdrop on a blade of grass. If
you find the experience pleasant, see if you can open fully to it.

Allow yourself to notice things you may ordinarily miss and to experience them fully. The warmth of the sun on your face, the wind in your hair, or whatever it might be.

You can use all of your senses, as appropriate: sight, smell, taste, touch, and sound. Stay with the experience until it feels complete for you, then open again to see what draws your attention next. Sense your environment and allow yourself to savor any positive experiences.

When the timer goes off, take a moment to reflect on what you noticed and how this compares to how you usually go about your life. Often we find we are more engaged with our lives. We realize what we've been missing while living our lives on autopilot.

When we share these experiences with another person, there is an opportunity for positivity resonance. Researcher Barbara Fredrickson, while studying the mechanisms of love, talks about love as a series of moments of positivity resonance. "Love is that micro-moment of warmth and connection that you share with another living being," she writes. These shared moments of positivity resonance over time are how we build a shared experience of well-being with others. We can actually use our own capacity to sense and savor positive experiences to build moments of positivity resonance with our partner. One practice I like is what I call the Partner Walk, which is based on an experience I had with mindfulness teacher Joanna Macy. If your partner is willing (or if you have a friend who is willing), give it a try.

TRY THIS
Partner Walk

As in the Sense and Savor Walk, we will be opening to positive experiences and savoring them, only this time sharing them with our partners.

Begin by finding a place you would like to explore that feels safe and is also one in which you both feel drawn to positive experiences.

Set a timer for a fixed amount of time, perhaps 5 minutes per partner. And determine who will be the guide and who will be the experiencer first.

If you are the experiencer, begin by closing your eyes. The guide then gently guides both of you as you walk along a path. When the guide sees something they are interested in—especially something they find pleasurable—they position you in front of the thing they find interesting. The guide can even gently position your head so that you will look right at whatever the guide has found. When both are ready, the guide says to you, "Open your eyes and see."

You, the experiencer, then open your eyes and take in whatever the guide has pointed you toward. Take a moment to savor the experience. There is no need to talk about the experience. It is often much more powerful when done in silence. When the guide is ready to move on, you close your eyes again, and the guide gently and carefully guides you to the next experience, carefully positioning you and inviting you to "Open your eyes and see." This continues until the timer goes off and then partners switch roles.

Note: As with all exercises and practices, it is important to customize this practice according to the needs of both partners. For example, it may be too much for some people to have their eyes closed while being guided. That's okay; the experiencer can simply keep a downward gaze until directed to open their eyes and see.

When both of you have had a chance to guide and experience, take some time to discuss what you saw together and your experiences of this practice. How is it to see through your partner's eyes? Beyond those moments of positivity resonance, it's helpful to practice taking in your partner's perspective. We often learn something we didn't know about our partners. For example, one couple living in a cold environment did this practice inside their own home. The husband was surprised to discover how much his wife loved their stove.

When we notice and savor the good in our lives, it often gives way to gratitude and appreciation.

Gratitude and Appreciation

Beyond these practices of sharing positive experiences, we can open to gratitude for the blessings in our life, including our partners' good qualities, and we can offer them our appreciation.

Gratitude

The practice of gratitude has been associated with better mental health and better relationships—even if the gratitude isn't shared. Because of the overwhelming evidence in support of the benefits of gratitude, many therapists recommend their patients keep a gratitude journal. At a set time, often before bed, patients are instructed to record three to five things they are grateful for.

This practice can also help correct the negativity bias in our relationships when we apply it to our partner.

TRY THIS

Gratitude for Your Partner

Audio Track 25

Often there are small things your partner does that you fail to notice, but from which you benefit. Maybe they bring you coffee, or take care of the bills, or laugh at your corny jokes. It could be something they've done for you, or it could be some quality they show that you really appreciate. Beyond the obvious things for which you are grateful, this practice provides the opportunity to practice seeing and appreciating the small things about your partner that can so often go unnoticed.

Please take out five pieces of paper and write on them:

What I appreciate about you is _____.

When this happens, I feel _____.
Thank you.

Or create a digital document and print out five copies. Leave plenty of space for what you might want to enter in the blanks.

Please allow your eyes to close, if that is comfortable, and bring your attention inward. You might notice the sensation of breathing or the sensation of hearing sounds. You might just notice the sensation of the body resting on the cushion or chair.

Now call to mind your partner. This imperfect being who has done things, especially small things, for which you are grateful.

What about your partner are you grateful for, especially small, tangible things that you often take for granted or over-look, like the way they often seem to have dinner ready for you, smile when they see you, help you with technology, are kind to your friends and family. Or the way your partner looks at you when you're having a hard time.

Notice how each thing makes you feel when it happens. Fill in the blanks on one sheet of paper for each thing you appreciate about them.

Notice how you feel compared to 10 minutes ago? That's the power of gratitude to generate positive emotions and to build intimacy.

It's likely that even though you haven't expressed your gratitude out loud to your partner you are already feeling closer, just by stopping to notice your partner's good deeds and good qualities. If you found this practice helpful, imagine how a regular practice of gratitude toward your partner could benefit you. If you like, you can keep a daily gratitude journal. Each evening (or whenever your set time is) you can take a few moments to record three things you are grateful for in your life and three things about your partner for which you are grateful.

Appreciation

Beyond cultivating gratitude, which often results in good feelings and goodwill in the person practicing gratitude, there is an opportunity here for the cultivation of love through positivity resonance. When we share what we notice and appreciate about our partners with them, we can land together in their good qualities and their impact on us.

Blocks to Appreciation

While sharing these notes of appreciation can make you feel vulnerable, receiving them can make some people feel even more vulnerable. Many of us are taught to deflect compliments. In fact, in teaching self-compassion around the world, it's the one thing I found every culture thinks is unique to them. When we discuss self-appreciation or opening to our own good qualities, they say something to the effect of "You don't understand. In our culture we have something called _____, and it means it isn't good to be full of yourself." It may be a different word in each culture, but it seems to exist in all of them.

At the heart of this aversion to being "full of ourselves" is often our desire to belong. If we think being seen as having particularly good qualities will somehow separate us from others or make us a target for them, we will, of course, resist the compliment.

However, common humanity says otherwise. Just as it is human to suffer (we all struggle sometimes), it is also common to have strengths. It doesn't make us different from others; rather it is also a condition of being human. We may not have the same strengths as others, just as we may not have the same suffering, but we do all have strengths.

> If you fear that being "full of yourself" will separate you from and make you a target for others, remember that just as we all struggle, we all have strengths too.

For others, it wasn't safe to be seen as having good qualities, especially in their family of origin. Perhaps you were met with "Who do you think you are?"

or people called you a princess or other derogatory terms. Or maybe you were punished or otherwise hurt when people close to you couldn't tolerate knowing your strengths. When this is the case, knowing our good qualities can activate the trauma pathway. We open our hearts to receive the compliment, and the pain of having been harmed is activated. When this happens, we become frightened at the thought of receiving compliments. Still, just as with backdraft, over time it is possible to rewire. We can learn to soak in appreciation just as we can learn to soak in compassion. It takes time, and we need to go very slowly.

Practicing Partner Appreciation

I mention these things because it can feel great to have your heart full of gratitude and to express it to your partner. However, if your partner is uncomfortable receiving compliments, you'll need to moderate the intensity of offering your appreciation so that it is a positive experience for both of you, rather than a traumatic one for your partner. Ways to decrease the intensity, when needed, are keeping the appreciation short (even one word), not making eye contact, and smiling and just saying thanks when you catch her doing something you appreciate or passing her a note of appreciation rather than saying it out loud—both are low-intensity ways to appreciate your partner. You can even leave a note for your partner to discover later, if that helps. If this is the case for your partner, you'll want to have a conversation with her about what she needs, if possible. Or you'll need to observe your partner to see which form she is comfortable with.

Others, however, have been craving appreciation and feel like they've gone years in the desert without water. They long for as much appreciation as you can give them. And sometimes they can't take in a simple thank you when you say it casually. Those people really need it to be special. The following exercise can help.

TRY THIS
Partner Appreciation

This exercise has two parts: offering appreciation and receiving appreciation. If your partner is willing to try the exercise with you, you can begin by doing the Gratitude for Your Partner exercise on page 243. Then you'll take turns offering appreciation and receiving appreciation. You can set a timer for 5 minutes each to practice this formally. However, if you don't have a partner willing to try this exercise with you, you can still try both parts of the exercise—appreciating and receiving—though they likely won't happen together and you'll have to be alert for when your partner (or someone else) happens to offer you appreciation in order to try the receiving part.

Offering Appreciation

With your gratitude notes from the gratitude exercise, take a moment to settle yourself by tending to your breath or doing whatever you like to become present in the moment.

Then turn your attention toward your partner. Consider how important your partner is to you and the things you are grateful for. Notice especially the impact their kindness has had on you and the good qualities or character traits behind their kind actions.

When you feel ready, please offer them your appreciation in whatever way is both heartfelt for you and comfortable for your partner. (This is the time to modify the practice as discussed above, if needed.)

As you let your partner know what you appreciate (for example, bringing you coffee in the morning), please let your partner know the impact those actions have on you. Then consider and name any good qualities in your partner that this kind action points to. An example would be:

"I love the way you bring me coffee in the morning. When you do, I feel loved and important to you. It also makes me appreciate your capacity for kindness. Thank you!"

It can also be helpful to hand your partner the note of gratitude you created for them.

If you are doing this practice with your partner in a formal way, you'll want to set a timer for about 5 minutes to let you know when your turn is over. You can keep naming things you appreciate about your partner until the timer goes off.

If you are doing this practice in an informal way with your partner, please watch your partner to see how they are doing with receiving the appreciation. As long as it appears to be a positive experience for both of you, feel free to offer as much appreciation as feels right to you. When you notice resistance or discomfort in your partner, it is likely a signal that they've had enough. In this case, less is more and more is less. You can offer more appreciation at another time.

When it is your turn to receive (either because the timer went off and you switched roles or because your partner happens to be saying thank you to you), see if you can let the compliment in fully. As best you can, open to receiving your partner's thanks and notice (or imagine) how that made your partner feel. Take pleasure in having made your partner feel good.

Then notice what good qualities in you allowed you to do something kind for them. As best you can, see if you can take that in too. Remember that we all have good qualities we show from time to time—that just makes us human.

When we can both express and receive appreciation with our partners, we can land in a state of positivity resonance. These are the micro-moments of love. Really knowing what has a positive impact on you is likely to increase your partner's motivation to try. Nothing breeds success like success. Landing in appreciation together can really create an upward relational spiral.

Awe

Another opportunity for positivity resonance is awe. Researchers have identified awe as a pathway to compassion. One definition of awe (from Dacher Keltner at the Greater Good Science Center) is "the feeling we get in the presence of something vast that challenges our understanding of the world, like looking up at millions of stars in the night sky or marveling at the birth of a child. When people feel awe, they may use other words to describe the experience, such as wonder, amazement, surprise, or transcendence."

We can share a moment of awe with our partners when we watch a beautiful sunset or when we spend time in the redwood forest and we see the size of these gentle giants. These are definitely moments of positivity resonance. The Partner Walk is a great way to open to experiences of awe together.

We can also feel awe at another person. Perhaps we are amazed by someone's artistic abilities or capacity for kindness. I've often been in awe when a patient or a participant in a class I'm teaching articulates something profound about his experience. I literally get goosebumps. There is a pause for me, and I don't want to say too much. Often the only thing I can say is "*Wow.* So beautifully articulated. Thank you." As my colleague Chris Germer says, "Saying anything more is like adding paint to Rembrandt."

There is something powerful in basking in the beauty of another person, especially when that person is your partner. It's hard not to be reminded of how much we love them or, if we were on the receiving end, how much we're loved and valued. To be seen by our partners in a positive light and recognized for our positive qualities fosters a sense of safety and belonging in the relationship. There is nothing better than being loved and appreciated for who we are.

> Basking in the beauty of another person, especially your partner, is very powerful.

Play and Joy

There is a saying, "The family that plays together stays together." Often we get so overwhelmed by the responsibilities of life that it is easy to put off seemingly optional things like play. Play is essential to our well-being. It lightens the load we carry when we allow ourselves the freedom to have some fun together. Playing together increases bonding, communication, conflict resolution, and relationship satisfaction.

Some studies have even found that having fun together is the most important factor in the sense of friendship and commitment, and the greatest influence on overall marital satisfaction. Do you remember what you used to do together? Is there a lighthearted spirit of playfulness in your relationship? One secret to remembering to practice compassion together is to make the practice fun. For example, in the Compassion for Couples (CFC) program, we help couples come up with personalized loving-kindness wishes they can share with each other. One way to lighten up that practice and make these wishes more accessible is to work with stones.

My partner and I collected stones from the local beach and wrote words (or you can draw pictures or symbols) on them that represented kind wishes for each other—things like love, confidence, rest, ease, and joy. The idea is to share the stones with each other informally whenever the urge strikes. We like to have a little fun with them by being a bit mischievous. For example, we may slip a stone or two into the other's suitcase before a trip. Or we may slip one under the other's pillow, to be found at bedtime. The wishes are genuine, and there is a sense of play and ease about offering them to each other.

This is a practice we also teach in the CFC program, and I've been impressed with how other couples have customized the fun for themselves. One couple wrote their wishes on poker chips. Another participant secretly wrote words on her husband's golf balls. He was quite moved (and his golf buddy was envious) when he pulled the balls out to use in his game and found the kind wishes written on them. No word on whether the wishes had any effect on his golf game.

When we open to our partners with a sense of playfulness and share activities that we find enjoyable, our happiness multiplies. Perhaps these activities reflect the core relational values you identified in Chapter 9. Which ones overlapped? Was it family, adventure, or exercise? Activities that honor those core values are likely to be both meaningful and enjoyable. They are a gift to you, your partner, and your relationship. Please make time for play and joy.

Being in a relationship requires we be there for each other in good times and in difficult times. We've spent most of the book exploring how to build a foundation of caring that will support us when difficult times inevitably arise and looking at how to navigate those difficult times with wisdom and compassion. Luckily that isn't the whole story. Making time for, opening to, and savoring those good times keeps that foundation strong. Love has many faces.

I love this poem by Julia Fehrenbacher, which expresses how love leads to a downpour of gifts:

Hold Out Your Hand

Let's forget the world for a while
fall back and back
into the hush and holy
of now

are you listening? This breath
invites you
to write the first word
of your new story

your new story begins with this:
You matter

you are needed—empty
and naked
willing to say yes
and yes and yes

Do you see
the sun shines, day after day
whether you have faith
or not
the sparrows continue
to sing their song
even when you forget to sing
yours

stop asking: *Am I good enough?*
Ask only
Am I showing up
with love?

Life is not a straight line
it's a downpour of gifts, please—
hold out your hand

Getting your mojo back as a couple often requires intentionally cultivating **more joy**. These shared experiences of joy, together with the capacity to weather difficult times with compassion, form the basis for a loving relationship. As noted in Chapter 1, while couples were offering each other their kind wishes in our workshop, Chris Germer remarked, "This is the *real* making love."

Remember that what you practice grows stronger. I hope you've learned helpful tools to get your relationship back on track or to keep it healthy if things are going well. Keep practicing. You matter. Your relationship matters. This is only the beginning of your new story. Keep going.

Resources

Books

Baraz, J., & Alexander, S. (2012). *Awakening joy*. Berkeley, CA: Parallax Press.

Brach, T. (2003). *Radical acceptance: Embracing your life with the heart of a Buddha*. New York: Bantam.

Brach, T. (2013). *True refuge*. New York: Bantam Books.

Brach, T. (2021). *Trusting the gold*. Louisville, CO: Sounds True.

Brown, B. (2015). *Daring greatly: How the courage to be vulnerable transforms the way we live, love, parent, and lead*. New York: Penguin Random House.

Chödrön, P. (1997). *When things fall apart: Heart advice for difficult times*. Boston: Shambhala.

Chödrön, P. (2002). *Comfortable with uncertainty*. Boulder, CO: Shambhala.

Chödrön, P. (2020). *Welcoming the unwelcome: Wholehearted living in a brokenhearted world*. Boulder, CO: Shambhala.

Cullen, M. (2015). *Mindfulness-based emotional balance workbook: An eight-week program for improved emotional regulation and resilience*. Oakland, CA: New Harbinger.

Dalai Lama [Tenzin Gyatso]. (1995). *The power of compassion*. New York: HarperCollins.

Fehrenbacher, J. (2021). *Staying in love*. New York: CCB Publishing.

Fredrickson, B. (2013). *Love 2.0: Finding happiness and health in moments of connection*. New York: Plume.

Germer, C. K. (2009). *The mindful path to self-compassion*. New York: Guilford Press.

Germer, C. K., & Neff, K. (2019). *Teaching the mindful self-compassion program*. New York: Guilford Press.

Gilbert, P. (2009). *The compassionate mind*. Oakland, CA: New Harbinger.

Gilbert, P., & Choden, P. (2013). *Mindful compassion: Using the power of mindfulness and compassion to transform our lives*. London: Constable & Robinson.

Gottman, J., & Silver, N. (2015). *The seven principles for making a marriage work: A practical guide from the country's foremost relationship expert*. New York: Crown.

Halifax, R. J. (2008). *Being with dying: Cultivating compassion and fearlessness in the presence of death*. Boston: Shambhala.

Halifax, R. J. (2018). *Standing at the edge: Finding freedom where fear and courage meet*. New York: Flatiron Books.

Hanh, T. N. (1998). *Teaching on love*. Berkeley, CA: Parallax Press.

Hanson, R. (2009). *The Buddha's brain*. Oakland, CA: New Harbinger.

Hanson, R. (2011). *Just one thing: Developing a Buddha brain one simple practice at a time*. Oakland, CA: New Harbinger.

Hanson, R. (2014). *Hardwiring happiness*. New York: Harmony Books.

Hanson, R. (2018). *Resilient*. New York: Harmony Books.

Hanson, R. (2020). *Neurodharma: New science, ancient wisdom, and seven practices of the highest happiness*. New York: Harmony Books.

Harris, D. (2014). *10% happier*. New York: HarperCollins.

Harris, R., & Hayes, S. (2008). *The happiness trap: How to stop struggling and start living*. Boston: Trumpeter Books.

Hayes, S. C., Strosahl, K. D., & Wilson, K. G. (2012). *Acceptance and commitment therapy* (2nd ed.): *The process and practice of mindful change*. New York: Guilford Press.

Hickman, S. (2021). *Self-compassion for dummies*. Hoboken, NJ: Wiley.

Johnson, S. (2008). *Hold me tight: Seven conversations for a lifetime of love*. New York: Hachette.

Kabat-Zinn, J. (1990). *Full catastrophe living*. New York: Dell.

Kornfield, J. (1993). *A path with heart*. New York: Bantam Books.

Kornfield, J. (2008). *The art of forgiveness, loving-kindness, and peace*. New York: Bantam Books.

Kornfield, J. (2008). *The wise heart*. New York: Bantam Books.

Kornfield, J. (2017). *No time like the present*. New York: Atria.

Neff, K. (2011). *Self-compassion: The proven power of being kind to yourself*. New York: William Morrow.

Neff, K. (2021). *Fierce self-compassion: How women can harness kindness to speak up, claim their power, and thrive*. New York: Harper Wave.

Neff, K., & Germer, C. (2018). *The mindful self-compassion workbook*. New York: Guilford Press.

Nepo, M. (2020). *The book of awakening* (20th anniv. ed.). Newburyport, MA: Red Wheel Publishers.

Nye, N. S. (1995). *Words under the words: Selected poems.* Portland, OR: Eighth Mountain Press.

Pollak, S. M. (2019). *Self-compassion for parents: Nurture your child by caring for yourself.* New York: Guilford Press.

Pollak, S. M., Pedulla, T., & Siegel, R. D. (2014). *Sitting together.* New York: Guilford Press.

Rosenberg, M. (2015). *Non-violent communication: A language of life.* Encinitas, CA: Puddle Dancer Press.

Salzberg, S. (1997). *Lovingkindness: The revolutionary art of happiness.* Boston: Shambhala.

Salzberg, S. (2011). *Real happiness: The power of meditation.* New York: Workman.

Salzberg, S. (2017). *Real love: The art of mindful connection.* New York: Flatiron Books.

Treleaven, D. (2018). *Trauma-sensitive mindfulness: Practices for safe and transformative healing.* New York: Norton.

Tutu, D., & Tutu, M. (2014). *The book of forgiving: The fourfold path for healing ourselves and our world.* New York: HarperCollins.

Podcast

Well Connected Relationships
https://wisecompassion.com/podcast
Together with guests who are experts in the fields of mindfulness, compassion, and relationships, I explore topics related to the intersection of compassion and relationships.

Websites

Center for Compassion and Altruism Research and Education, Stanford
http://ccare.stanford.edu

Center for Mindful Self-Compassion
https://centerformsc.org

Center for Mindfulness (Basel, Switzerland)
https://zentrum-fur-achtsamkeit.ch

Center for Mindfulness (Finland)
https://mindfulness.fi

Center for Mindfulness, University of California at San Diego
https://cih.ucsd.edu/mindfulness

Center for Mindfulness and Compassion, Cambridge Health Alliance,
Harvard Medical School Teaching Hospital
https://chacmc.org

Compassion for Couples, Wise Compassion
https://wisecompassion.com

Compassion Cultivation Training (CCT), Compassion Institute
https://compassioninstitute.com

Compassion Focused Therapy, Compassionate Mind Foundation (UK)
https://compassionatemind.co.uk

Compassion It
https://compassionit.com

The Couples Institute Counseling Services (San Francisco Bay area)
https://couplesinstitutecounseling.com

The Gottman Institute
https://gottman.com

Greater Good Magazine, Greater Good Science Center at UC Berkeley
https://greatergood.berkeley.edu

Institute for Meditation and Psychotherapy
https://meditationandpsychotherapy.org

The Mindfulness Network (Iceland)
https://home.mindfulness-network.org/tag/iceland

The Mindfulness Project (UK)
https://londonmindful.com

Notes

Foreword

PAGE X: **The curious paradox:** Carl R. Rogers. (1995). *On becoming a person: A therapist's view of psychotherapy.* New York: Houghton Mifflin. (Original work published 1961)

PAGE XI: **Every marriage is a mistake:** quoted in Frank S. Pittman & Tina Wagers. (2005). The relationship, if any, between marriage and infidelity. *Journal of Couple and Relationship Therapy, 4,* 135–148.

Chapter 1. We All Need to Be Loved

PAGE 17:   **The role of oxytocin and attachment in parent–child relationships:** J. E. Swain et al. (2014). Approaching the biology of human parental attachment: Brain imaging, oxytocin and coordinated assessments of mothers and fathers. *Brain Research, 1580,* 78–101.

PAGE 19:   **The role of caring for a plant in the health of seniors:** Emily J. Nicklett, Lynda A. Anderson, & Irene H. Yen. (2016). Gardening activities and physical health among older adults: A review of the evidence. *Journal of Applied Gerontology, 35*(6), 678–690.

PAGE 19:   **Therapeutic alliance and positive outcomes in psychotherapy:** John C. Norcross. (2011). *Psychotherapy relationships that work: Evidence-based responsiveness.* New York: Oxford University Press.

PAGE 19:   **Touch and reduction of pain:** P. Goldstein, I. Weissman-Fogel, & S. G. Shamay-Tsoory. (2017). The role of touch in regulating inter-partner physiological coupling during empathy for pain. *Scientific Reports, 7*(1), 3252.

PAGE 20: **Poetry by Naomi Shihab Nye:** *Words under the words: Selected poems.* (1995). Portland, OR: Far Corner Books.

PAGE 22: **The importance of "turning toward" in relationships:** J. Gottman & N. Silver. (2015). *The seven principles for making marriage work: A practical guide from the country's foremost relationship expert.* New York: Crown.

PAGE 23: **Self-compassion and relationships:** Kristin D. Neff & S. Natasha Beretvas. (2013). The role of self-compassion in romantic relationships. *Self and Identity, 12*(1), 78–98.

PAGE 23: **Secure attachment in families:** Yoo Rha Hong & Jae Sun Park. (2012). *Korean Journal of Pediatrics, 55*(12), 449–454.

PAGE 23: **Benefits of a secure bond ripple outward:** Sue Johnson. (2008). *Hold me tight: Seven conversations for a lifetime of love.* New York: Hachette.

PAGE 24: **Compassion in work teams:** *Understand team effectiveness.* Project Aristotle. Available at *https://rework.withgoogle.com/print/guides/5721312655835136.*

PAGE 24: **The role of a strong back and a soft front:** Roshi Joan Halifax. (2008). *Being with dying: Cultivating compassion and fearlessness in the presence of death.* Boston: Shambhala, p. 18.

PAGES 26-27: **Survival of the most cooperative:** E. Pennisi. (2005). How did cooperative behavior evolve? *Science, 309*(5731), 93.

Chapter 2. "Why Can't You Be Here for Me?": Understanding What Gets in the Way

PAGE 32: **Negative emotions narrow our focus:** Barbara L. Fredrickson. (2001). The role of positive emotions in positive psychology: The broaden-and-build theory of positive emotions. *American Psychologist, 56*(3), 218–226.

PAGE 32: **Velcro for negative emotions, Teflon for positive emotions:** Rick Hanson. (2020). *Neurodharma: New science, ancient wisdom, and seven practices of the highest happiness.* New York: Harmony Books.

PAGES 32-33: **Affect regulation systems:** Paul Gilbert & Kunzang Choden. (2015). *Mindful compassion: Using the power of mindfulness and compassion to transform our lives.* London: Constable & Robinson.

Chapter 3. "I Wish I Could Fix It!": Resisting Pain with Problem Solving

PAGES 42-43: **Emotion contagion, empathy, and compassion:** Tania Singer & Olga M. Klimecki. (2014). Empathy and compassion. *Current Biology, 24*(18), R875–R878.

PAGES 43-44: **The drive system:** Paul Gilbert & Kunzang Choden. (2015). *Mindful compassion: Using the power of mindfulness and compassion to transform our lives.* London: Constable & Robinson.

Chapter 4. "Do You Care?": Finding Safe Connection

PAGES 61-63, 72-75, 77-78: **The care system, soothing, and affiliation:** Paul Gilbert & Kunzang Choden. (2015). *Mindful compassion: Using the power of mindfulness and compassion to transform our lives.* London: Constable & Robinson.

PAGE 63: **Avenues for connection:** J. E. Steller, A. Cohen, C. Oveis, & D. Keltner. (2015). Affective and physiological responses to the suffering of others: Compassion and vagal activity. *Journal of Personality and Social Psychology, 108*(4), 572–585.

PAGES 63-64: **Touch and pain reduction:** Pavel Goldstein, Irit Weissman-Fogel, Guillaume Dumas, & Simone G. Shamay-Tsoory. (2018, March 13). Brain-to-brain coupling during handholding is associated with pain reduction. PNAS, *115*(11), E2528–E2537.

PAGE 64: **Therapeutic presence and therapeutic alliance in psychotherapy:** Shari M. Geller. (2017). *A practical guide to cultivating therapeutic presence.* Washington, DC: American Psychological Association.

PAGES 64-68: **Strong back and soft front:** Kristin Neff & Christopher Germer. (2018). *The mindful self-compassion workbook: A proven way to accept yourself, build inner strength, and thrive.* New York: Guilford Press.

Kristin Neff. (2021). *Fierce self-compassion: How women can harness kindness to speak up, claim their power, and thrive.* New York: HarperCollins.

PAGE 69: **The importance of "turning toward" in relationships:** J. Gottman & N. Silver. (2015). *The seven principles for making marriage work: A practical guide from the country's foremost relationship expert.* New York: Crown.

PAGES 68-69: **On the courage of vulnerability and relationships:** Brené Brown. (2015). *Daring greatly: How the courage to be vulnerable transforms the way we live, love, parent, and lead.* New York: Penguin Random House.

Chapter 5. "Who Will Love Me?": Ensuring That Compassion Is Always Available to You

PAGES 84, 96: **Research on self-compassion and how we treat others:** Christopher Germer & Kristin Neff. (2019). *Teaching the mindful self-compassion program: A guide for professionals.* New York: Guilford Press.

PAGES 84-85, 87-88, 90: **Three components of self-compassion:** Kristin Neff & Christopher Germer. (2018). *The mindful self-compassion workbook: A proven way to accept yourself, build inner strength, and thrive.* New York: Guilford Press.

PAGES 92-94, 96: **Mindful Self-Compassion:** Christopher Germer. (2009). *The mindful path to self-compassion: Freeing yourself from destructive thoughts and emotions.* New York: Guilford Press.
Kristin Neff. (2011). *Self-compassion: The proven power of being kind to yourself.* New York: William Morrow.

PAGE 92: **The power of touch:** D. Keltner. (2009). *Born to be good: The science of a meaningful life.* New York: Norton.

PAGES 94-95: **Mindfulness and the window of tolerance:** David Treleaven. (2018). *Trauma-sensitive mindfulness: Practices for safe and transformative healing.* New York: Norton.

Chapter 6. Being Present: Mindfulness Skills to See Clearly and Quiet Reactivity

PAGE 101: **Mindfulness and the three components of self-compassion:** Kristin Neff & Christopher Germer. (2018). *The mindful self-compassion workbook: A proven way to accept yourself, build inner strength, and thrive.* New York: Guilford Press.

PAGES 104, 107-115: **Mindfulness practices:** Jon Kabat-Zinn. (2013). *Full catastrophe living: Using the wisdom of your body and mind to face stress, pain, and illness.* New York: Bantam Books.

PAGE 110: **Mindfulness and the window of tolerance:** David Treleaven. (2018). *Trauma-sensitive mindfulness: Practices for safe and transformative healing.* New York: Norton.

PAGE 114: **The attitude of generosity:** Brené Brown. (2015). *Daring greatly: How the courage to be vulnerable transforms the way we live, love, parent, and lead.* New York: Penguin Random House.

PAGES 115-116: **On the courage of vulnerability and relationships:** Brené Brown. (2015). *Daring greatly: How the courage to be vulnerable transforms the way we live, love, parent, and lead.* New York: Penguin Random House.

Chapter 7. Cultivating Connection: Strength in Common Humanity

PAGES 125-126: **Common humanity and the three components of self-compassion:** Kristin Neff & Christopher Germer. (2018). *The mindful self-compassion workbook: A proven way to accept yourself, build inner strength, and thrive.* New York: Guilford Press.

PAGE 128: **The story of Procrustes:** Jean Shinoda Bolen. (2014). *Gods in everyman: Archetypes that shape men's lives.* New York: Harper-Collins.

PAGES 136-137: **Ubuntu:** Claire E. Oppenheim. (2012). Nelson Mandela and the power of ubuntu. *Religions, 3,* 369–388.

Chapter 8. Getting What We Need: Kindness in Three Directions

PAGES 149-150, 152, 155-156, 158-161, 169: **Caring force, the spectrum of self-kindness, and the components of compassion:** Kristin Neff & Christopher Germer. (2018). *The mindful self-compassion workbook: A proven way to accept yourself, build inner strength, and thrive.* New York: Guilford Press.

Christopher Germer & Kristin Neff. (2019). *Teaching the mindful self-compassion program: A guide for professionals.* New York: Guilford Press.

Christopher Germer. (2009). *The mindful path to self-compassion: Freeing yourself from destructive thoughts and emotions.* New York: Guilford Press.

Kristin Neff. (2011). *Self-compassion: The proven power of being kind to yourself.* New York: HarperCollins.

Chapter 9. "What Really Matters to Us?": Rooting Your Relationship in Your Values

PAGE 176: **Values versus goals:** S. C. Hayes, K. D. Strosahl, & K. G. Wilson. (1999). *Acceptance and commitment therapy: An experiential approach to behavior change.* New York: Guilford Press.

PAGES 187–188: **The role of core values:** R. Harris & S. Hayes. (2008). *The happiness trap: How to stop struggling and start living.* Boston: Trumpeter Books.

Chapter 10. "How Can We Really Get Each Other?": Using Compassionate Communication Skills

PAGE 189: *Nonviolent communication:* Marshall B. Rosenberg. (2015). *Nonviolent communication: A language of life.* Encinitas, CA: Puddle Dancer Press.

PAGES 192–193: **Emotion contagion, empathy, and compassion:** Tania Singer & Olga M. Klimecki. (2014). Empathy and compassion. (2014). *Current Biology, 24*(18), R875–R878.

PAGE 194: **Unsolvable relationship problems:** Michael Fulwiler. (2012). Managing conflict: Solvable vs. perpetual problems. Available at *www.gottman.com/blog/managing-conflict-solvable-vs-perpetual-problems.*

PAGES 197–198: **Mark Nepo excerpt:** Mark Nepo. (2020). *The book of awakening* (20th anniv. ed.). Newburyport, MA: Red Wheel Publishers.

Chapter 11. "Can We Heal Our Wounds?": Cultivating the Conditions for Forgiveness

PAGES 217, 219–220: **On forgiveness:** Desmond Tutu & Mpho Tutu. (2014). *The book of forgiving: The fourfold path for healing ourselves and our world.* New York: HarperCollins.

PAGE 220: **"Forgiveness is not forgetting":** M. Cullen. (2015). *Mindfulness-based emotional balance workbook: An eight-week program for improved emotional regulation and resilience.* Oakland, CA: New Harbinger.

PAGE 221: **Well Connected Relationships podcast:** M. Becker (Host). (2020, November 30). Forgiveness with Margaret Cullen (No. 7) [Audio podcast episode]. In *Well Connected Relationships.* Available at *https://wisecompassion.com/podcast.*

Chapter 12. "How Do We Keep Our Love Alive?": Celebrating Positive Experiences Together

PAGE 238: **The magic ratio:** J. Gottman & N. Silver. (2015). *The seven principles for making marriage work: A practical guide from the country's foremost relationship expert.* New York: Crown.

PAGES 239-240: **Taking in the good:** Rick Hanson. (2016). *Hardwiring happiness: The new brain science of contentment, calm, and confidence.* New York: Harmony Books.

PAGES 241, 245, 248: **Positivity resonance:** Barbara L. Fredrickson. (2013). *Love 2.0: Finding happiness and health in moments of connection.* New York: Plume.

PAGE 251: **"Hold Out Your Hand":** Julia Fehrenbacher. (2021). *Staying in love.* New York: CCB Publishing.

Index

About the Author

Michelle Becker, MA, LMFT, a marriage and family therapist in private practice in San Diego, is dedicated to helping people thrive in healthy, well-connected relationships. She is the developer of the Compassion for Couples program and cofounder of Wise Compassion (*www.wisecompassion.com*). She is also a cofounder of the teacher training program at the Center for Mindful Self-Compassion and a senior teacher of Compassion Cultivation Training. Through workshops, online education, and a podcast, she shares the knowledge and tools required for people to relate to each other better.

Track	Title	Run time
1	Finding Strength and Softness	5:25
2	Uncovering Your Survival Strategies and How They Impact Your Partner	5:52
3	Discovering Our Tendencies to Fix and Finding Vulnerability Underneath	4:57
4	Discovering What's Underneath Your Need to Control, What Your Partner Feels, and How to Speak from Vulnerability	3:29
5	Finding the Strong Back of Compassion	3:57
6	Finding the Soft Front of Compassion	4:31
7	Discovering How We Treat Ourselves and Others	5:35
8	Putting Self-Compassion into Practice with Mindfulness, Common Humanity, and Kindness	8:54
9	Supportive Touch	4:31
10	Soles of the Feet	4:10
11	Awareness of Breath	7:41
12	Awareness of Sound	5:38
13	STOP	5:35
14	Touching Hands	5:06
15	Discovering Common Humanity	5:57
16	Belonging	6:48
17	Loving-Kindness for Couples	9:13
18	Motivating Yourself with Compassion	12:22
19	Soften, Soothe, and Allow	8:42
20	Meeting Our Own Needs	4:47
21	Discovering Your Core Values	5:16
22	STOP and LOVE	13:43
23	Forgiving Others	7:48
24	Forgiving Yourself	7:22
25	Gratitude for Your Partner	3:51